Praise for
Explorations of a Mind-Traveling Sociologist

"*Explorations of a Mind-Traveling Sociologist* is like reading a story of a life and a story of a soul at the same time. In her beautifully written and enriching book, Renée Fox is engaged and engaging, deeply curious and informed, clear thinking and open-minded, humane and compassionate. She is as much a teacher as she is a scholar, and she is always a listener. What a joy to read such a wise and insightful book of life and living."
—The Reverend Peter Kountz, Vicar, Saint Stephen's Episcopal Church, Philadelphia, USA

"Eye-opening, gripping and utterly engaging ethnographic essays from one of the great minds of our time. The book stands as testimony to the power of the human mind and the transcendence of the human heart and spirt. People are seen in their humility and frailty—but also in their nobility and strength. A must-read for anyone seeking understanding of life or uplift of spirit."
—Kenneth M. Ludmerer, Professor of Medicine, Professor of History and the Mabel Dorn Reeder Distinguished Professor of the History of Medicine, Washington University, St. Louis, USA

"Rightly revered as a pioneering figure in both the Sociology of Medicine and Bioethics, Renée C. Fox, now in her 90s, here offers her many readers an elegant collection of essays that are both personal and ethnographic. Whether writing about the staff in her apartment building or about the heroic efforts of Doctors Without Borders to deal with the outbreak of Ebola, Fox displays a novelist's eye for detail and a social scientist's eye for context, as she leads the reader outward from the seemingly narrow world of her near confinement, due to her advanced age and frailty, and into the wider world of medicine and politics with which she remains actively engaged and deeply connected. In doing so, *Explorations of a Mind-Traveling Sociologist* foregrounds and highlights Fox's deepest value commitments and the ideals that have guided her work from *Experiment Perilous* to *Doctors Without Borders*: the determination to break free of the 'social boxes' of her origins and to develop an empathetic understanding of the experiences and sufferings of others.

Ultimately, *Explorations of a Mind-Traveling Sociologist* is a confession of faith: faith in the liberating and illuminating potential of cross-cultural research into the lived experience of others; faith in the goodness of a life devoted to the calling of the scholar-teacher; and faith in the goodness of those devoted to ministering to and witnessing the suffering of others. As such, this book is a gift both to Fox's many admirers and to future generations of her readers."

—Howard L. Kaye, Emeritus Professor of Sociology,
Franklin and Marshall College, Lancaster, PA, USA

"Renée Fox, an indefatigable and gracious nonagenarian scholar, casts her experienced sociological gaze near and far, sharing intimate thoughts about her personal life, and perspicacious observations on local, political and more distant global events. These 'emerita essays' augment her prodigious scholarly output that place her in the pantheon of legendary sociologists."

—Solomon Benatar, Emeritus Professor of Medicine,
University of Cape Town, South Africa

"Renée Fox shines with 'amazing grace': in her way of looking at the world around her, in her relationships with people, in her writing. Reading her leads to a state of equanimity rarely encountered in the social sciences."

—Yves Winkin, Emeritus Professor, Urban Anthropology,
University of Liège, Belgium

"Renée C. Fox has been a worldwide traveler and explorer of social relations over the many decades she spent doing ethnographic research in the sociology of medicine. How then does someone who has qualified herself as a perpetual fieldworker sustain that activity when the frailties of age and disability limit her mobility? *Explorations of a Mind-Traveling Sociologist* testifies to the persistent vitality of Fox's instinct to explore, whether it be by reflecting on her past travels and research as they are embodied in her home surroundings and as they are regularly brought up to date by her continued connection with those she has met in the field, in the classroom or simply in her everyday surroundings. Unlike the memoir she published some years ago whose aim was to recount her life, *Explorations of a Mind-Traveling Sociologist*, a mosaic of essays on persons, problems and events encountered over the years, highlights her value commitments and points to the challenges she feels will require our most urgent attention."

—Simone Bateman, Emeritus Senior Researcher, CNRS
(National Center for Scientific Research), France

"Renée Fox is internationally renowned for her insightful, phenomenological analysis of life on the personal, scientific and geographic frontiers of medicine. For much of her life, her keen reflections arose from first-hand observations in hospitals, clinics and research centers in Africa, Europe and the United States. Though no longer able to explore the world, she has now produced the ne plus ultra of her remarkable career in this wonderful book, with its fresh, intercutting examinations of her seven decades of amazing experiences and encounters that have a lot to say about the world today."

—A. M. Capron, University Professor, University of Southern California, and First Director, Ethics, Trade, Human Rights, and Law, World Health Organization

"Renée C. Fox invites us to join her as a participant observer as she 'mind travels' across the globe, exploring issues from outbreaks and immigration to humanitarian crises and bioethics. Renée inspires us to be everyday sociologists, questing and advocating for meaningful solutions to some of society's most pressing problems."

—Peter Piot, Director, London School of Hygiene & Tropical Medicine, UK

"Aging has finally done to Renée Fox what war, disease, discrimination against women and other obstacles could not. Renée can no longer travel to Europe, Africa and China to conduct her groundbreaking ethnographic research, but the elegant essays in this book show that she is still exploring her world."

—William Whitworth, Editor Emeritus, *The Atlantic*

"One of twentieth century's leading sociologists continues to write with deep insight, empathy and force. My first contact with Fox's writing was in 1984, when my life was redirected by her 1963 essay on how doctors are trained for 'detached concern.' I became her student in 1989 and then really saw her extraordinary mind and essayistic power up close. She has been a constant teacher, by her words and example, to countless people in all walks of life. And she is still teaching, with joy. In *Explorations of a Mind-Traveling Sociologist*, each subtle observation opens into a whole world of ideas—about living with constraints, about humanitarian medicine, about contested elections, about the art of teaching itself."

—Nicholas A. Christakis, Sterling Professor of Social and Natural Science, Yale University, New Haven, CT, USA

Explorations of a
Mind-Traveling Sociologist

Renée C. Fox

Foreword by
Anne Fadiman

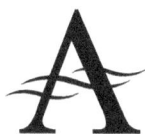

ANTHEM PRESS

Anthem Press
An imprint of Wimbledon Publishing Company
www.anthempress.com

This edition first published in UK and USA 2020
by ANTHEM PRESS
75–76 Blackfriars Road, London SE1 8HA, UK
or PO Box 9779, London SW19 7ZG, UK
and
244 Madison Ave #116, New York, NY 10016, USA

British Library Cataloguing-in-Publication Data
A catalogue record for this book is available from the British Library.

Library of Congress Cataloging-in-Publication Data
Library of Congress Control Number: 2019952770

ISBN-13: 978-1-78527-142-7 (Hbk)
ISBN-10: 1-78527-142-3 (Hbk)
ISBN-13: 978-1-78527-145-8 (Pbk)
ISBN-10: 1-78527-145-8 (Pbk)

This title is also available as an e-book.

This book is dedicated to the persons who throughout the course of my professional lifetime as a sociologist I have been privileged to teach; to those who have made it possible for me to conduct firsthand ethnographic research in the United States, Europe, Africa and Asia, accompanying me in the process; and to the companion coauthors and editors who enabled some of the fruits of my teaching and research to be published in meaningful prose.

CONTENTS

Part 5: On Being a Teacher

FOREWORD
Anne Fadiman

What if you were a great sociologist who had devoted your life to fieldwork that had taken you all over the world: to Europe, where you had investigated the social and cultural aspects of Belgian medical research and listened to carillon bells ringing from Gothic belfries; to Central Africa, where you had traced the development of the Congolese medical profession and walked through streets littered with broken glass from the Simba Rebellion; to China, where you had observed how Deng Xiaoping's Four Modernizations policy played out in a Tianjin hospital and delivered a lecture to the Chinese Academy of Medical Sciences in an auditorium so cold that the entire audience wore padded jackets and long underwear; to South Africa, where you had studied the strategies employed by Médecins Sans Frontières to combat the HIV/AIDS pandemic and attended a mass rally for antiretroviral treatment at which hundreds of Gugulethu residents sang and danced in the rain; and to dozens of other countries where you had conducted research in medical ethnography as a participant observer? And what if, because of age and physical frailty, you were now largely confined to your apartment? What would you do?

Most people would throw in the towel and feel their lives were over. Renée Fox is not most people. Even though her outer landscape has radically contracted, what she calls her "inner landscape" is so expansive that her travels are far from ended. Her current mode of conveyance is her mind. At 91, she is still a participant observer; she is still doing fieldwork; she is still, in Clifford Geertz's terminology, "thickly descriptive," though the subject of her thick description is now often her own daily life. The essays in this book are the product of her inextinguishable ethnographic curiosity, which allows the near to summon the far, the inward to summon the outward, the present to summon the past.

Renée lives in an elegant apartment off Rittenhouse Square in Philadelphia that is filled—but not cluttered—with books, maps, photographs and art, most of it connected in one way or another to her half-century of international research. The world comes to Apartment 1103/4 in the form of phone calls, emails, cards and letters from her academic colleagues, her fieldwork collaborators and, especially, her former students, who continue to view her as a source of seer-caliber counsel. She keeps up with current affairs, especially in the medical sphere, not only through newspapers, radio, and television but through updates from friends who work with Médecins Sans Frontières. From time to time a troop of Penn medical students with an interest in writing—members of the Gawannabes, so called because, secretly or not-so-secretly, they all aspire to be Atul Gawande—blow in, along with a whoosh of millennial fresh air, to tell her about their experiences in the anatomy lab and the surgical theater.

I teach writing, and on the first day of class, when I talk about the virtues of concision, I always quote from a Wordsworth sonnet called "Nuns Fret Not at Their Convent's Narrow Room." The topic of the poem is constraint. Wordsworth tells us that just as nuns accept their cramped quarters and bees enjoy the slender foxglove bells in which they gather nectar, so do poets value the sonnet's enforced brevity and strict rhyme scheme. From narrow rooms come great things: prayer, honey, literature.

Unlike the nuns and the bees and the poets, Renée Fox has not chosen her life's constraints. The fates have handed her an existential deal that is both kind and cruel: superlative mind, compromised body. She would doubtless prefer that her leg, her arm, and her ribs had not been broken by falls; she would doubtless prefer not to use the walker necessitated by post-polio syndrome; she would doubtless prefer a less narrow room.

But dealing with constraints—or, to be more exact, refusing to be constrained by constraints—has been a recurring theme throughout Renée's life. Polio at 17? She took a year off from Smith to recover and rehabilitate, then returned to graduate summa cum laude. Limited academic opportunities for women sociologists in the 1950s? After completing her doctorate at Harvard (though with a diploma from Radcliffe, since women were not yet permitted to receive Harvard degrees even after following the same curriculum as their male classmates), she initially received no teaching offers, so she accepted a research position at Columbia before becoming a tenured faculty member at Barnard, chairing the sociology department at Penn, and being inundated by a Niagara of medals and prizes, including a knighthood: the Chevalier de l'Ordre de Leopold II, conferred by the Belgian government. Too young and too female to be a likely candidate for a Guggenheim Fellowship—not to mention that Guggenheims were rarely granted to sociologists? She applied anyway, at 32, and of course she got one.

I might add that although Renée routinely refuses to take no for an answer, the refusals are always tendered with consummate politeness. The word "lady" has fallen into disrepute of late, but Renée is a lady in the best sense of the word. My favorite photograph in her apartment—it's part of the montage on the cover of this book—is of her walking in the copper mines of Katanga with her friend Willy De Craemer, the Jesuit priest with whom she collaborated on much of her research in the Congo. She is wearing a chic dress, a chic scarf, and chic pumps. In 2010, Renée and I found ourselves at a Harvard commencement together, I as a member of one of the university's governing boards and she to receive an honorary degree. Female Overseers traditionally wear white gloves to commencement. Renée immediately noticed that mine were … I blush to say it … *nylon*. It wasn't long before a package arrived at my home containing two exquisite pairs of gloves, one silk, one leather.

By that time, Renée and I were good friends. We had met 11 years earlier, when I became the editor of *The American Scholar*, a literary quarterly to which she was a contributor and on whose editorial board she served. I particularly enjoyed editing a piece she wrote about the year she had spent as the 57th George Eastman Visiting Professor at Oxford. (Of the previous 56, 55 had been men.) It wasn't just a memoir, it was an *ethnography*, in which, among other things, she analyzed the hierarchy of the Balliol College Fellows as indicated by whether or not they had been allotted silver napkin rings. (She had.)

A few months before the nylon-glove commencement, Renée called to discuss Bill Whitworth, an editor who had worked with me at *The American Scholar* and edited Renée's autobiography, *In the Field*. Over the years, Renée and I had both exchanged innumerable emails and had innumerable phone conversations with Bill, but he worked from his home in Arkansas, and neither of us had met him. Renée believed this situation demanded a remedy, and she proposed one: we would fly to Little Rock and take Bill out to dinner. She was 82 at the time, and although not yet housebound, she moved with difficulty. But this was one of those instances in which Renée was not going to take no for an answer. We had a wonderful time.

As I read the essays collected in *Explorations of a Mind-Traveling Sociologist*, I thought of something the Belgian novelist Jan-Albert Goris had said when Renée was 34 and had just published an article in *Science* that shone an affectionate but high-wattage light on some of the more problematically traditional aspects of his country's culture. Whether or not one agreed with Renée Fox, remarked Goris, "she has *moed*." *Moed* is the Flemish word for courage. Renée Fox still has *moed*.

PREFACE

When my book *Doctors Without Borders: Humanitarian Quests, Impossible Dreams of Médecins Sans Frontières* was published in 2014, I knew it was destined to be the last book of this sort I would write.[1] I was still in fundamentally good health and blessed with lucidity, but because of the aging of my body and the post-polio symptoms it was manifesting, I could no longer undertake the physically strenuous ethnographic research in the array of American, European, African and Asian settings that underlay my *Doctors Without Borders* book and characterized my research throughout my career.

Journeying into the field as a questing sociologist and writing about what I had learned and come to understand through the participant observation it involved were so vital to my being that it was hard for me to imagine a life, much less a book, without them. Slowly, however, the idea for a feasible book that contained these elements began to take shape: a book of thematically interconnected ethnographic essays drawn from a range of things I was seeing, experiencing, thinking and feeling at this juncture in my life, whose participant observer outlook would extend its purview beyond autobiography or memoir.

***

Composing these essays has been an engrossing undertaking. It has heightened and enriched the observations that I make in the course of my daily life. It has enabled me to engage in "mind travel" to places I have intimately known in the past and to places I have yearningly hoped to visit but never have.[2] It has strengthened my connectedness with persons who have been important presences in my life—among whom figure prominently persons I have taught over the years and persons who helped me conduct the field research in which I was involved. And in fulfilling my continuing need to write, I have

---

[1] Baltimore: Johns Hopkins University Press.
[2] I am indebted to Anne Fadiman for describing my nonphysical travel as "mind travel."

experienced what the Israeli author David Grossman has described as "the great miracle, the alchemy" of this act:

> In some sense, from the moment we take pen in hand or put fingers to keyboard we have already ceased to be at the mercy of all that enslaved and restricted us before we began writing.
>
> We write. How fortunate we are: The world does not close in on us. The world does not grow smaller.[3]

* * *

A friend with whom I shared my plan to write this book characterized its essence as "observations and analyses from your apartment, with a window on the world outside and inside." It is from that perspective that these essays begin with an unexpected incident in my apartment.[4]

---

[3] David Grossman, "Writing in the Dark," in *Writing in the Dark: Essays on Literature and Politics*, trans. Jessica Cohen (London: Bloomsbury, 2008), p. 68.

[4] In this book, when quoting from email messages and other correspondence, I have altered names and other identifying characteristics to protect the identity of many of my correspondents.

ACKNOWLEDGMENTS

I am deeply indebted to all of the individuals whose background, personal stories, professional training and histories, value commitments and resonant voices constitute the substance of this book of ethnographic essays. They include family members, friends, colleagues, students and former students and health professionals, many of whom appear in the book, who have been integral to the meaningfulness of my past and present life and who have helped me function on an everyday level at this elderly, physically restricted phase of my existence. These persons also include the staff of the apartment house in which I have dwelt for decades, and the home health aides who more recently have enabled me to continue to live in my apartment, surrounded by my library, my files of firsthand field notes and my personal and professional memorabilia.

Notwithstanding all the support and help I have received in the course of writing this book, it would never have found its way into print without Jacqueline ("Jackie") Wehmueller, whom I first came to know when she was executive editor at Johns Hopkins University Press, where she shepherded my previous book about Doctors Without Borders and me through the publishing process. She has played an even more encompassing role with regard to this book—including the many nuanced ways she has edited its text, the generosity and skill with which she has facilitated my communication with Anthem Press and the constant, uplifting encouragement she has bestowed on me.

In addition, the vibrant, dedicated group of persons who have knowingly and unknowingly, explicitly and implicitly, contributed to the coming into being of this book consist of the following.

Anne Fadiman, the renowned essayist, writer of memoir and biography and of literary nonfiction and inspiring teacher of writing at Yale University, has graced this book with her preface and its author with her friendship.

Jonathan Imber, professor of sociology at Wellesley College, and editor-in-chief of the journal *Society* (whose PhD dissertation I had the honor of directing many years ago), to whom I am profoundly indebted for the indefatigable help he gave me in searching for and finding a publisher for this book.

Judith Watkins, research librarian, who with efficiency and graciousness did the tediously meticulous work that was involved in obtaining permissions for the use of all the firsthand verbatim quoted data in the book.

The medical historian Judith P. Swazey, who has been my partner as a coinvestigator and coauthor in connection with a great deal of the sociological field research I have conducted, and the articles and books based upon it that I have published. So much has this been the case that we were dubbed "the team of two" by some of our research informants and respondents in the People's Republic of China. What is more, over the years, my relationship with Judith became one of deep and encompassing kinship not only with her but also with her husband, Peter, her son, Peter ("Woody"), and her daughter, Beth—who is my goddaughter. Judith read many of the essays in this book in their early drafts and, as always, improved them with candidly astute criticisms and suggestions.

Olga Shevchenko, professor of sociology at Williams College, whose research, teaching and publications are centered in postsocialist Russia, and who was my companion participant observer and my mentor in the research on the activities of Doctors Without Borders in Russia in which I was engaged.

Tovia Freedman, whose doctoral training in social work has involved her in conducting clinical consultations with members of the branches of the US military service and their families in Europe and Asia, as well as in the United States, and in the care of hospice patients, and who, along with her husband, William Freedman, acted as a first responder to the 9/11 terrorist attacks.

William Freedman, emeritus professor of electrical and computer engineering at Drexel University, with expertise in issues associated with postural sway and its effects on the stability of stance in the elderly and with cervico-ocular reflex and vestibulo-ocular reflex effects on the eye.

Mark Gould, professor of sociology at Haverford College, a committed, intellectually challenging and creative social theorist, and a dedicated, stimulating teacher.

Mary Ann Meyers, a scholar, teacher and writer in the field of American civilization, who served as secretary of the University of Pennsylvania and president of the Annenberg Foundation and is presently a trustee of the John Templeton Foundation.

Carole Joffe, professor of sociology emerita at the University of California, Davis, whose research, writing, teaching and advocacy have focused on reproductive health, with special attention to abortion provision.

Judith Brown, historian of India and Modern South Asia, Oxford University professor emerita and an ordained Anglican priest.

Peter Kountz, former head of the Charter School of Architecture and Design (CHAD) in Center City, Philadelphia, and presently an Episcopalian priest who is the vicar of Saint Stephen's Episcopal Church in Philadelphia.

Neville Strumpf, a nurse-scholar and pioneering leader in the nursing care of elderly persons, emerita professor of gerontology at the University of Pennsylvania School of Nursing and its interim dean emerita, and a member of the advisory board of the Barbara Bates Center in the History of Nursing.

Jan Jaeger, who began her career as a registered nurse in surgery and emergency medicine at Thomas Jefferson University and went on from there to study at the University of Pennsylvania, where she obtained a degree in healthcare management at the Wharton School of Finance and a PhD in sociology. Among her significant professional roles have been manager of the US Navy's Department of Human Research Protection and of the Institutional Review Board of Operations at Harvard University, and her ongoing position as the chief human research consultant for the Population Studies Center at the University of Pennsylvania.

Kenneth Ludmerer, a physician and historian, distinguished professor of medicine and history at Washington University in St. Louis, who has spent his professional lifetime studying the evolution of academic medicine and medical education in the United States. His renowned books include *Let Me Heal*, *Learning to Heal* and *Time to Heal*.

Deborah Frank, professor of pediatrics and director of the Grow Clinic for Children at Boston Medical Center, who is the founder and principal investigator of Children's HealthWatch, a network of pediatric and public health researchers working to improve child health, and a highly respected national authority and eloquent public advocate with regard to the growing problem of hunger and its effects on children in the United States and to the effects of intrauterine exposure to cocaine and other substances on children's long-term development.

Robert Klitzman, professor of clinical psychiatry at the College of Physicians and Surgeons and the Mailman School of Public Health at Columbia University, who is the cofounder of the Columbia University Center for Bioethics, director of Columbia's master's in bioethics program and former director of the Ethics and Policy Core of Columbia's HIV center. He is a gifted and prolific author who has published numerous books based on in-depth, thickly descriptive, firsthand qualitative data which deal with the processes and experiences of becoming a physician and a psychiatrist (including physicians' experiences when they become patients), the spiritual needs of patients, the lives of men and women with HIV, genetic testing, "designing babies" and the struggle to make human research safe. He is also the prolific author of op-ed pieces that are relevant to his medical, ethical and social expertise, commitments and concerns.

Solomon ("Solly") Benatar, emeritus professor and head of the Department of Medicine at the University of Cape Town, emeritus chief physician of the Groote Schuur Hospital, past founding director of the University of Cape Town Bioethics Center and annual visiting professor in medicine and public health sciences in the Dalla Lana School of Public Health at the University of Toronto. In addition, he has been an invited lecturer at medical schools throughout the world and has published hundreds of articles and book chapters on a wide range of topics that include respiratory medicine, academic freedom, medical ethics and the humanities in medicine, human rights, health-care systems, health economics and global health. Wherever he travels, Solly and his wife, Evelyn ("Evie"), remain in close touch with me, and whenever they are in Toronto, I receive weekend telephone calls from them that nostalgically remind me of the calls I received every Sunday from my parents during my youth.

Throughout the time it has taken me to write this book, I have been supported, and skillfully and devotedly cared for medically, by my primary care physician, Dr. Lillian Cohn; doctor of physical medicine and rehabilitation Keith Robinson; and physical therapist Gail Kotel—supplemented recently by periodic discussions with psychiatrist Marc Inver.

A team of home health aides that includes Alzie Henry, Keyonia Renton, Breanna McCleary and Eleanor Ripley has enabled me to live safely and function capably within my apartment—especially in the wake of a recent fall that resulted in several painful, debilitating fractures.

Unobtrusively, but faithfully, my sister and brother-in-law, Rosa and Robert Gellert, have caringly and constantly watched over me, as has their grandson, Leopold Spohn-Gellert—my grandnephew—whose uplifting visits and company I greatly appreciated and enjoyed during his years as an undergraduate at the University of Pennsylvania. In addition, with subtle concern, my sister-in-law Geraldine ("Gerry") Fox has maintained steady, comforting contact with me through her weekly telephone calls.

These are the persons who have helped make it possible for me to write and complete this book. I am very fortunate—and profoundly thankful to them.

Part 1

APARTMENT NUMBER 1103/4

Chapter 1

RESILIENCE

The last days of September and the first days of October this year have been uncommonly cold, grey and rain-soaked. The central heating system has not yet been turned on in my apartment house. (The landlord is not legally obliged to do so until October 15.) Even when I don a jacket that would ordinarily be appropriate for outdoor wear, I shiver from the chilliness that permeates my home.

Inexplicably, late in the evening on October 1, I fell as I was walking toward my study where I was intending to work a little longer on the draft of an essay I was writing. I was helped back on my feet by the person on duty at the main desk of the apartment house, whom I reached by phone to ask for assistance. I was not injured by the fall, although I did sustain a few bruises. But I was thrown off balance by it, emotionally as well as physically. I no longer felt confident about the techniques of cautious walking that I have developed, or the safeguards such as grip bars and flat, wall-to-wall carpeting that I have installed in the apartment, to protect me from falling. And I was too shaken to resume writing.

* * *

I awoke the next morning to an eruption of news concerning a mass shooting the previous day by a 26-year-old gunman in a classroom of Umpqua Community College in Roseburg, Oregon, that had killed 10 persons (including, by suicide, the perpetrator) and wounded 9 others. The story of this rampage was headlined on the front page of the *New York Times* and featured in dramatic detail on all the morning TV news programs.

A day later another kind of tragic, deadly event occurred—one that received international attention and media coverage. A trauma center hospital run by Doctors Without Borders/Médecins Sans Frontières (MSF) in Kunduz, Afghanistan, was bombed from the air by a US military plane. Among those killed were 14 MSF staff members, 4 relatives of patients and 24 patients, including 3 children, while 37 people were injured, among whom were 19 members of the MSF team. I had reacted with horror to the lethal Oregon community college incident. But I was even more stricken and morally disturbed by the news of the hospital bombing, because it was an act that violated international humanitarian law under which hospitals in conflict zones are protected spaces, because of the role that an American gunship seemed to have played in transgressing this law and also because of my deep personal identification with MSF through my many years of firsthand research inside this medical humanitarian organization and movement.

* * *

In the days that followed I contacted several members of MSF with whom I have especially close relations. I wanted to express the shock, sorrow and indignation that I felt in the wake of the hospital bombing, to obtain more information about the damage and casualties it had involved, to seek an explanation of how and why it had happened and to ask whether there was anything I could do to be helpful. The answers that came back referred to the bombing as "a dark page" in MSF's history which was part of "an ongoing silent tragedy" that revealed "what civilians endure on a daily basis in Afghanistan, and even more so now in Syria, under the term 'collateral damage.'" They characterized the bombing as an "absurd" as well as "inexcusable" happening, especially because during the past 10 years MSF had spent a significant amount of time talking to the United States and other countries about the need to protect their health facilities, particularly in Afghanistan where, since the opening of their hospital in Kunduz in 2011, they had "treated tens of thousands of wounded civilians and combatants from all sides of the conflict." What was called for now, in the words of the statement made by Dr. Joanne Liu, the international president of MSF, that one of my contacts sent me before it appeared in the press, was "a transparent, independent investigation" of the airstrike: "This attack does not just touch MSF, but it affects humanitarian work everywhere, and fundamentally undermines the core principles of humanitarian action. We need answers, not just for us but for all medical and humanitarian staff assisting victims of conflict, anywhere in the world."[1]

* * *

---

[1] "MSF: Dr Joanne Liu says MSF denounces blatant breach of International Humanitarian Law," *Polity*. https://www.polity.org.za/print-version/msf-dr-joanne-liu-says-msf-denounces-blatant-breach-of-international-humanitarian-law-2015-10-06

It is now October 12. I am still moving about in my apartment with greater wariness and anxiety than before my recent fall. But my apprehension has diminished. It is not only the passage of time that accounts for this. It is also the enduring impact that the shooting episode in an American community college and the bombing of a hospital in Afghanistan have had on me, which have put in perspective the perils that I face in my sheltered existence—how minor and delimited they are in comparison to such violent catastrophes. I have been energized by the indignation that I have felt in the wake of what happened in Roseburg, Oregon, and in Kunduz, Afghanistan, to which I have been transported in my mind, and uplifted by the responses that members of MSF shared with me. As a consequence, I have been able to resume writing—an activity essential to my sense of purpose and meaning—from which this essay has emerged.

Chapter 2

APARTMENT NUMBER 1103/4

Within my spacious apartment, number 1103/4, where I spend more time as I age and become less mobile, the past, the present, the succession of generations and the future coexist in objects, in books and documents, and in images. What they embody extends beyond the apartment and the views outside its windows to all the places in the world where my work has carried me. I am vitally linked to those places not only in memory but also through the immediacy and import of the messages my international correspondence brings me—like the email I received when I began drafting this essay, from a friend who is a member of the international medical humanitarian organization Doctors Without Borders:

> Am on my way flying back [from the Central African Republic] to South Africa while writing this […] As you can imagine, Ebola is on everyone's mind down there, up to the most remote part of the country, while they expect some cases to come […] from the Democratic Republic of Congo. I strongly hope it will not happen to that already devastated country.

Apartment number 1103/4 is composed of two identical smaller apartments that were merged long before I moved into it in 1980, a decade after becoming a professor at the University of Pennsylvania. It is on the 11th floor of a 16-story, pre–World War II residential building in Center City, Philadelphia, close to Rittenhouse Square, one of the city's small open-space parks planned by William Penn in the late seventeenth century.

At the center of the apartment is my large and serene study, where I spend many of my long waking hours. During the day, even in inclement weather, the study is illumined by the light that penetrates its six surrounding windows. It is encircled by floor-to-ceiling bookcases, filled with hundreds of colorful books—neatly aligned, topically organized.

Adjacent to my well-used Herman Miller desk, on a shelf below two of the study's windows, an electric typewriter occupies an honored place. It is the

IBM Selectric II on which I composed all my manuscripts and the letters that I did not handwrite before I made a reluctant transition to computer. Near it sits a Rolodex file in which I stored addresses typed on index cards in my pre-computerized days.

Despite the proficiency that I have attained in using a computer, I still have a wary relationship with it. Whenever it behaves in ways that perplex me—which is often—I need not only technical assistance but also a modicum of supportive therapy, usually provided by Jeff Katz, my on-call computer expert. Jeff can access my computer from his, remotely diagnosing and fixing some of the problems I encounter. If working directly on my computer seems to be called for, he obligingly makes a home visit. Jeff visits my apartment frequently—mainly because although I have some agility in using my computer, I understand very little about how it works and am often too perplexed by the problems that arise to effectively describe them to Jeff, much less fix them on my own.

Recently Jeff came to my apartment on a Saturday morning to help me deal with my computer mouse. His wife and his 10-year-old daughter came with him on this visit, because they planned to have lunch together in a Center City restaurant. When he had dealt with my mouse, Jeff walked his daughter over to look at my IBM Selectric typewriter. He uncovered it, pointed out its component parts and explained how it worked. She gazed at the typewriter and listened to what her father was saying about it as if it were an intriguing museum exhibit, which in fact it was for her, since she had never seen a typewriter. For me this incident dramatically captured the magnitude of technological change that has occurred over the course of my lifetime. How antique some of the artifacts of my existence seem to a girl who is 78 years younger than I am.

Carefully and sentimentally arranged in the study are memorabilia from some of the places where my research and teaching have transported me over the years. Among them are a small replica of *The Adoration of the Mystical Lamb*, the early fifteenth-century Flemish altarpiece in the chapel of St. Bravo's Cathedral in Ghent painted by Hubrecht and Jan van Eyck; a *matryoshka* Russian nesting doll, carved by a homeless man living on the streets of Moscow who received aid from Doctors Without Borders; a map of the Democratic Republic of Congo constructed of cobalt and malachite extracted from the country's mines; and a framed watercolor portrait of the Belgian dramatist Michel de Ghelderode, who, in his antique penmanship, inscribed in French on its reverse side these words: *For Renée Claire Fox—wounded angel with tender eyes … a flame that the wind can curve, but extinguish, no ….*[1]

---

[1] For an account of my relationship to de Ghelderode, see "'Les Roses, Mademoiselle!' The Universe of Michel de Ghelderode," in Renée C. Fox, *In the Belgian Château: The*

There are also photos of persons whose entwined personal and professional presence in my life has had the deepest significance for me: my foremost teacher and mentor, the sociologist Talcott Parsons; medical historian Judith Swazey, my sisterly friend, coinvestigator, coauthor, and her children, Beth and Woody; and Willy De Craemer, a sociologist, Jesuit priest and nonproselytizing missionary, for whom sociological research and teaching were a calling. It was Willy, as I once wrote, who "made it possible for me to travel to places inside and outside of myself that I would never have known otherwise [including to the heart of Africa], and who [...] understood the sense of my life better than anyone else."[2]

There is a photo of the anthropologist Margaret Mead in the study, too. I was not her student in the conventional sense of the term. But she took note of me, and made things happen for me professionally at a critical point in my career, in a way that exemplified her active interest in the potentialities and aspirations of young social scientists.

On the wall across the room from my desk, above the cobalt-and-malachite map of the Congo, I have placed a yellowing Japanese flag that is attached to a bamboo pole. Printed on the flag, Japanese characters spell out congratulations: "Welcome for having climbed Mount Fuji, 3,776 meters." Willy De Craemer received it in recognition of his summiting Mount Fuji, Japan's highest mountain. Every time I look up from my desk and gaze across the room, I see that flag. It is emblematic for me of Willy's global vision, and of his physical, emotional and moral courage throughout the progressive phases of Parkinson's disease that eventuated in his death.

Hanging below the flag and the map is a recent addition: a framed certificate that looks much like a diploma and officially states that "Renée C Fox has been duly elected as a Fellow National [sic] of The Explorers Club, given under our hand and seal on the 25th of January 2014"—signed by the president and the secretary of the club. I placed it there because it seemed to me to be related to what the Congolese map and the Japanese flag stand for. But in certain respects it is also an anomaly—a document pertaining to what I initially considered one of the most unlikely honors ever bestowed on me.[3]

Spirit and Culture of a European Society in an Age of Change (Chicago: Ivan R. Dee, 1984), pp. 181–204.

[2] See the dedication to my ethnographic autobiography, Renée C. Fox, *In the Field: A Sociologist's Journey* (New Brunswick, NJ: Transaction Publishers, 2011), and the chapters titled "Africa, Léopoldville, Kisantu, and Usumbura," "My Years in the Congo," and "Willy's Last Days," pp. 159–200 and 397–408.

[3] See "Election to the Explorers Club" herein.

Closer to my desk is a cluster of photos—including one that Beth and Woody Swazey had taken together and put in a frame embossed with "We Love You" on its perimeter, a snapshot of my sister and brother-in-law, Rosa and Robert, and within a silver frame, on whose rim is etched "In Friendship" and the date 2008, a group picture of those who joined me and each other to celebrate my 80th birthday. In addition, there is a photograph of two young Japanese girls, standing in front of the bookshelves in my study, playing a duet for me on their violins. In the course of a trip they made to the United States with their mother, a sociologist whom I taught when I was a visiting scholar at Tokyo Medical and Dental University, they spent an afternoon in my apartment. Their mother arranged their musical performance for me, and took the picture.

On the left-hand wall of the study near the hall hangs a large framed photograph of the front gate of the 2,000-bed general hospital in Kinshasa, shaded by tall palm trees and surrounded by women draped in colorful cotton *pagnes*, wearing kerchiefs or turbans, carrying babies on their backs and bundles on their heads, men with bicycles, and several male medical staff members clad in white coats. In the mid-1960s, when this picture was taken and I did my first stint of research in the Congo, Kinshasa was known as Léopoldville, and the hospital had no particular name. But during the second interlude of my research in that area in the 1970s, under the presidency of Mobutu Sese Seko and his policy of African "authenticity," Léopoldville had been renamed Kinshasa, the Congo, Zaïre, and the hospital became the *Hôpital Mama Yemo*, in honor of Mobutu's mother.

Above the photo of the hospital, framed in a cinematic sequence, is a series of snapshots of Willy De Craemer and me walking amid the excavations of a copper mine in the Congo's Katanga Province. Willy is dressed in a tropical white cassock which, in the days before the Second Vatican Council, constituted the everyday wear of Catholic priests working in sub-Saharan Africa. My own appearance in these photos amuses me every time I glance at them. The image that I see is that of a woman some fifty years younger than I am now, with an earnest, inquiring expression on her face, who looks incongruously modish in that setting. Her long hair is coiffed in a smooth pageboy, over which she has arranged an attractive kerchief. She is clad in a fashionable (albeit decorous) summer dress, and she is wearing hose and pumps with Cuban heels. In those shoes I was able to walk with a less pronounced post-polio limp, and at that time—in the 1960s—it would have been considered improper in the Congo for a woman to wear pants rather than a dress or a *pagne*. But viewed from my current perspective, the way I am garbed in this snapshot seems comical.

* * *

When they enter the other rooms of my apartment, many visitors comment on its orderly immaculateness, and also, with some surprise, on the modernity of its furnishings. Most of the furniture, which I brought with me when I moved to Philadelphia in 1969, was designed in the 1950s and the early 1960s. It comes from a post-World War II era of modernism, an interior designer friend of mine informed me, that is now known as "mid-century modern." So, I guess there is a sense in which it could be considered to be rather antique modern. But, my friend says, it is a style that has come back into vogue and is enjoying a resurgence; as a consequence, its current value exceeds the modest prices I paid for it when, as a junior faculty member, I was earning no more than 10,000 to 12,000 dollars a year.

I asked my designer friend to make the rounds of my apartment with me and point out some of the pieces in it that have become vintage mid-century modern. In the dining room, he identified the burl-oak table on a chrome base, the four "T chairs" designed by William Katavolos surrounding it made of tan leather slung on three-legged chrome frames, and the "Sputnik"-style chrome chandelier with its 12 globe-shaped bulbs. In the living room, he singled out the tan leather armchairs, the orange velvet upholstered couch, the teak and aluminum wall system, the high-fidelity record player and the Scandinavian rug with its orange, gold and brown abstract pattern. In my bedroom, he paid particular attention to the clear Plexiglas pedestal chair that he said was a Laverne Tulip Chair, and to the pendant ceiling lamp, constructed of multi-colored metal shards.

But the personality and the spirit of my apartment do not reside primarily in my furniture. Rather, they emanate from certain images and objects — beginning with those in my study—by which I am surrounded.

One of the most arresting objects in the apartment is a huge, detailed, paper map of the city of Kinshasa that I brought back from the Congo and had mounted on a three-paneled screen. It dominates the dining room, which is adjacent to the study. Lining the dining room's walls, arranged in an art gallery–like way, is an *in seriatim* display of the abstract pastels and paintings that a Japanese artist friend of mine, Umeko Kato, created, and has sent to me over the years from Kitakyushu. Central to every one of them is a woman, represented by her face, one or more infants, the artist's relationship as a mother to those children, and her thoughts—depicted as a bird—about what being a woman and a mother entail.

Walking through the hallway brings me in contact with Belgium, the small European society that, beginning in 1959, I traversed for more than thirty years, initially to conduct a sociological study of Belgian medical research. That investigation progressively evolved into a study of Belgium through the windows of its medical laboratories, which in turn transported me to

Africa—to the former Belgian Congo (Zaïre/the Democratic Republic of Congo)—where from 1962 to 1970, I became deeply immersed in firsthand sociological research.[4] Enduring imprints that Belgium made on me are visible in what I have framed and hung on the corridor walls. There are four photographs of some of the hundreds of stone statues in canopied niches that cover the entire exterior of Leuven's Gothic town hall—statues of patricians, noblemen and personages of importance in that town's local history, and of patron saints. There is also a poster, issued at the time of the 1976 exposition held in Brugge (Bruges) to celebrate the 800th year of Sint-Janshospitaal (Saint John's Hospital), and its medical, artistic and religious importance through the centuries. The poster depicts an Augustinian religious sister associated with the hospital's historically famous pharmacy, dressed in a traditional nun's habit, compounding a medicine with a pestle in a waist-high ancient brass mortar.

In the hallway I grouped together two other framed Belgium-connected artifacts. One is the front cover of *In the Belgian Château*, the book that I published about my research in Belgium. The illustration on its jacket is a version of the Surrealist Belgian artist René Magritte's famous painting known as *Empire of Light* or *The Dominion of Light*, which paradoxically depicts the dark, nighttime exterior of a house illumined by only one small street light, under an azure blue, sunlit, daytime sky. Below the cover hangs the engraved certificate that, along with a medal, I received in 1975 "at the proposal of" the Belgian Minister of Foreign Affairs and "the royal decree" of the reigning King of the Belgians, Albert II, which conferred on me "a decoration in the Belgian National Orders in the rank of 'Chevalier [Knight] of the Order of Leopold II.'" In presenting me with this decoration, the then Belgian ambassador to the United States thanked me for writing such an "authentic and affectionate book about Belgium." I had discovered many things that even Belgians did not know about their country, he said, and identified other things of which they were aware but did not fully recognize or appreciate.[5] Whenever I pass by this document, whatever flicker of pride about it I may feel is instantly counterbalanced by my memory of what a little boy named Jake said when his mother, one of my former students, explained to him that the framed certificate on the wall he was looking at made me a knight. That isn't possible, he exclaimed with indignant certainty. "Only *men* can be knights!"

I don't know what Jake would have thought about the fact that only men were accorded Harvard University degrees in 1954 when I completed my PhD graduate study in sociology under the aegis of Harvard's Department of Social Relations. The diploma that I received at that time was a Radcliffe

---

[4] For an account of this research and its trajectory see Fox, *In the Belgian Château*.
[5] Fox, *In the Field*, pp. 339–42.

College one, countersigned by the president of Harvard. This was the primary reason that I decided to display on an adjacent corridor wall what I view as the diploma from Harvard that I *finally* received in 2010, when the university awarded me an honorary Doctor of Laws degree.

At the far end of the hall there is a door on which, with a combination of solemnity and whimsy, I have attached an elaborately lettered **ARCHIVES** sign that I had made for it. Behind the door is a small room that is lined on one side with tightly filled bookshelves and, on the other, with a row of three large metal files, four drawers high. The preponderance of books are associated with the subject of my most recently published book about Doctors Without Borders and global medical humanitarian practice and action. Placed on one of the topmost shelves, out of easy view, is a copy of each of the books that I have published over the years. The files contain meticulously organized and indexed field notes and primary and secondary documents associated with the research I have conducted, notes and syllabuses for the courses I have taught, manuscripts of lectures I have given, and reprints of articles I have published. Notably missing from these files are most of the field notes and documents related to my years of research in Belgium and in the Democratic Republic of Congo. The Belgian materials have been deposited in the archives of the Catholic University of Louvain in Louvain-la-Neuve, Belgium, and the Congolese materials in the Contemporary History Section of the Royal Museum of Central Africa in Tervuren, Belgium. The contents of the files in my archives room (along with those in several smaller files in other rooms of my apartment) have been accepted "for permanent preservation" by the Harvard Medical Library in the Francis A. Countway Library of Medicine in Boston. The library would be willing to receive those materials at any time, and for a while I considered the possibility of sending them to Boston as soon as I could pack them for shipping. But when I realized that inhabiting an apartment with empty files would make me feel desolate, I decided not to do so.

Humanizing the books and papers are the photos on the archive room's walls. There is a photo of Suzanne Mikanda, my long-ago research companion in the Congo, with whom, through correspondence that has spanned time and space, I have maintained a deep, familial relationship. "*Très chère Yaya*"—"Very dear Older Sister"—is how her messages to me begin. Hanging nearby is a photo of another close friend and colleague, pediatric surgeon and bioethicist Farhat Moazam, with the staff at the Centre of Biomedical Ethics and Culture in Karachi, Pakistan, that she founded and directs, and below it, a snapshot of one of her associates, sitting under an open red parasol that is sheltering him from a leak in the center's ceiling as he conscientiously types on his computer. In addition, there are photos of the children of two of my former students. In one of them, two little boys who are brothers have been posed by their mother with an open copy of my memoir *In the Field* in their hands, as though they were reading it together; and in the other, a little girl, flanked by her mother (now the chair of a college anthropology and sociology department, whom I taught during her graduate student years) and her father, is holding up a large crayon picture she has drawn, on which she has printed "Happy Birthday, Renée," in wobbly capital letters. And across the room, there is a formal wedding picture of a student I taught when she was an undergraduate, who has become a plastic surgeon.

I have also framed and hung on the walls of this room other recent honorary degrees I have received: a Doctor of Social Science degree from King's College in London in 2010, and in 2011, a Doctor of Science degree from the University of Pennsylvania. I have mixed feelings about having done so. Although I am grateful and proud to be their recipient, displaying both of them, in close proximity to each other, seems rather self-vaunting. In addition, it evokes complex questions for me concerning how much significance one should attach to such honors, and about how to deal with them in a respectful but non-egotistical and practical way. Certainly the solution is not to fill the walls with documents that flamboyantly attest to them! In my apartment, I have dealt with these questions by limiting the number of such honors that I exhibit, and by surrounding the two honorary degree diplomas in the archives room with photos of cherished former students, esteemed colleagues and their progeny to whom I attach unqualified, unambivalent importance.

And I am unambivalently proud of, and continually touched by, the poster I received as a gift from the staff of the Johns Hopkins University Press that I have hung on the door inside the archives room. Below the image of the cover of my book about Doctors Without Borders that is affixed to it, and encircling the "With Gratitude" message written in elegant script on its face, are the signatures of all the members of the press who were involved in the publication of the book.

Outside the door to the archives, on the right-hand wall, are two posters whose texts I cannot read, because one is printed in Chinese and the other in Japanese. They are notices of the series of public lectures that Judith Swazey and I gave in Tianjin, China, when we were there together in 1981, doing field research at the Tianjin Central Hospital,[6] and of the lectures that I delivered in 2011 when I was teaching at the Tokyo Medical and Dental University.

* * *

---

[6] For a narrative account of this research experience, see Fox, "China, 1981: Tianjin and the 'Team of Two,'" in Fox, *In the Field*, pp. 299–318.

The walls of the adjacent room (where visiting friends from out-of-town sleep on what I hope they experience as a comfortable sofa bed) are decorated with posters that are souvenirs of invited lectures I gave at Albert Einstein College of Medicine, Harvard Medical School, Smith College, Radcliffe College, the Université Catholique de Louvain and the Universiteit Katholieke Leuven. On the far side of this room are shelves filled with a mixed assortment of books. Among them, those that pertain to religion are the most abundant; a whole section of the shelves is reserved for books by former students and close colleagues. The contents of the two small and unobtrusive files in the room consist mainly of field notes from the many years of firsthand research on social, cultural and historical aspects of hemodialysis, organ transplantation and the development of an artificial heart in which Judith Swazey and I collaboratively engaged.

A recent addition to this room is a chair, the first piece of furniture I have purchased in many years. It does not fit with the sleek, artistically designed contours of the mid-century modern furniture that predominates in my apartment, or with the characteristically vivid colors of their accessories. Rather, it is a large, thickly padded chair, upholstered in a muted shade of blue, with a stuffed quilted back, wide armrests and big side pockets. Technically speaking, it is an electrically powered "lift chair," with an "autodrive hand control" that enables me to raise the entire chair up from its base, extend its footrest, and move it into various degrees of reclining positions. Such chairs are described in a Wikipedia entry as "useful to the elderly, infirm, or disabled" because they "can aid comfort and mobility and also provide independence." While I am elderly, I do not consider myself to be infirm. I am, however, disabled by the post-polio-associated weakness of some of my muscles, the torsion of my neck and the scoliosis of my spine. My physical therapist, who recommended that I acquire the chair, said that sitting and reclining in it would provide me with relaxation and respite from pain that would be diffusely beneficial.

Incorporating the chair into my daily rounds should be helpful. What is more, doing so would exemplify a maxim that I hear myself rather piously stating to others from time to time—namely, that although it may seem somewhat paradoxical, accepting various kinds of assistance can help one to become more independent. But the fact that I view this chair as less comely than the other furniture in my apartment, and that I have located it in a room that I only occasionally enter, suggests that to a greater degree than I have consciously admitted I regard it as a signpost on the road to greater dependency, down which I am moving with a complex mixture of trepidation, reluctance and defiance.

***

In that room, there is a closet where I keep a vacuum cleaner, an ironing board, bed linens, a laundry basket and spare hangers. It is also the place where I have stored three of the suitcases that accompanied me on some of my travels. Although they are empty and immobile now, they are silent witnesses to the trips we once shared, about which they tacitly remind me when I go into my closet.

In Spring 2016, the imminent blooming of Washington, DC's famed cherry blossoms and the pink and white blossoms on the dogwood and cherry trees in Rittenhouse Square Park were accompanied by an outburst of news from friends, colleagues and family members about their pending plans for travel to Europe, South America, Asia, and within the United States for sightseeing, teaching and relaxation.

The interest and pleasure that I have in hearing about these incipient and often far-ranging travels are comingled with pangs of nostalgia and feelings of regret. They evoke memories of all the journeying I have done in the course of my life, and the acute realization that due to my bodily impairments and advanced age I will never again be able to physically travel very far beyond my apartment and its environs.

* * *

Moving past this room and the archives room next to it brings one to the threshold of the living room. There is a stillness in this room that is remote from the study in which most of the social as well as intellectual activity in the apartment takes place. And an aura emanates from the African art objects housed within it. Most of those displayed on the shelves of the wall system were fashioned by artists of Kuba-Congolese origins. Kuba ethnic culture is renowned for its art, and all of the Kuba pieces in my living room—the wooden boxes, the wood- and ivory-sculpted human figures and the copper and wood machetes—are carved somewhere on their surface with beautiful, characteristically Kuba geometric patterns. An abstract image of a Congolese woman carrying a baby on her back and a pile of wood on her head, hammered out on a large copper plaque, hangs on the wall space between the two sets of shelves. And grouped on the large glass table in the center of the room, along with a free-form fragment of copper that I retrieved from the ground in Katanga, are several small wooden objects from the Equator region of the Congo, given to me by Suzanne Mikanda, who was born and grew up in this area, and who told me that they were associated with traditional, Ngombe tribe, magico-religious rituals.

Among the many persons who have viewed the African pieces in this room, very few have noticed that there is a distinctly non-African artifact I have mischievously placed in their midst. It is a pair of bronzed high-top laced shoes—the shoes in which I took my first steps as a baby. They were sentimentally preserved in this way for my parents by a company that existed during my childhood whose primary business consisted of baby shoe bronzing.

Unobtrusively located in a far corner of the living room is a small, built-in set of bookshelves, filled mostly with novels and with a poignantly impressive collection of books that my largely self-educated father purchased and read in his late teens and early 20s, after he left school because he felt a duty to work full time to help support his parents and siblings.

The most private room of the apartment, my bedroom, lies just beyond the living room. Although it is the apartment's most sequestered room, it has the only floor-to-ceiling windows that look out panoramically on the environing city streets and the surrounding skyline. Framed by those windows is a tall palm plant, reminiscent of my years in the Congo. The glass bedside table holds an ever-changing assortment of books that I am currently reading. The voluminous book on the table desk across the room occupies a permanent status here. It is an *Encyclopedia of New York City*—the city where I was born, where I grew up and where I taught for 11 years at Barnard College.

Every night, after I close the book I have been reading and switch off the lamp on my bedside table, I turn on my right side in preparation for falling asleep. When I do so, through my bedroom windows I see a broad pattern of illumined windows in a large apartment house located several blocks away from mine. I can approximate what time it is by the number of lights turned on in these dwellings. The more lights I see, the earlier it is in the evening; the more darkened windows there are, the later it is.

Two windows in particular have taken on a special meaning for me. One of them gleams especially brightly, and is among those that stay on the longest. The other is framed by a balcony that on certain nights is festooned with multicolored green, red and blue lights. It seems to me that it is especially on Friday evenings that those lights appear, and I wonder whether they have a weekend or Sabbath significance for the persons who light them. Inexplicably, I feel connected with the inhabitants of those two apartments, whoever they are. As I make the transition from being awake to falling asleep, I feel reassured by the presence of their lights, and something akin to regret if the lights are extinguished.

My bedroom is the room that contains the most photographs of my family and those who are like family to me. There are pictures of my mother and my father at various times in their younger years, including one of my mother in her 1920s flapper-style wedding gown; of my sister Rosa and brother-in-law Robert on a trip they made to Prague, Czechoslovakia, Robert's birthplace; of Judith Swazey, her late husband Peter, and their dachshund, Cognac, on the porch of their cabin in Maine; of Willy De Craemer as a pensive Flemish boy, later as a Jesuit seminarian, and subsequently as a priest, with and without his Roman collar; and the wedding photos of two of my former students.

There are two photographs of me among this gallery of photos. One of them, a smiling portrait of me as a six-month-old baby, lying on my stomach, naked, except for a diaper tied and buttoned around my bottom, is the center-piece of an advertisement for "Pynless Diapers" [*sic*], published in *Child Life* magazine, for which I was the model. This amusing, photo-illustrated adver-tisement that I inherited from my parents was framed and kept on perpetual display by them in the apartments we lived in during my childhood. The other picture of me was taken in a professional photographer's studio when I was four or five years of age. I am arrayed in a silk party dress of that era, with a large grosgrain ribbon bow in my hair, and I am gazing lovingly at the doll in my lap—a rag doll with long blonde curls, a purple coat and patent leather shoes, whom I remember naming "Cookie." I have hung alongside it a photograph of Mila, another little girl— the daughter of a sociologist I taught when she was a graduate student. Holding a doll that I gave her as a birthday present, Mila is looking at it with the same affectionate tenderness that is displayed in the comparable photo of me.[7]

The most transcendental image inside my bedroom is the first one I see when I awake in the morning and the last one I see at night before I turn off my bedside lamp. It is a detail from Fra Angelico's masterpiece *The Last Judgment*, painted by an anonymous copyist, that hangs above the table desk on the wall directly across from my bed. It depicts Paradise as a place where angels are leading the saved, two by two, hand in hand, through a beautiful garden into a shining city that they are entering. I don't know what Fra Angelico would say about how I interpret it. But for me it represents the ideal of being united forever with the most significant persons in one's life.

---

[7] The doll is a replica of "Eloise," the little girl who lived in a room "on the tippy-top floor" of the Plaza Hotel in New York. She is the main character in a series of children's books written by Kay Thompson and published by Simon & Schuster—the first of which was published in 1955.

Chapter 3

A HALLWAY FRIENDSHIP

My apartment, number 1103/4, is located at one end of the long hall on the 11th floor of The Wellington, the building in Philadelphia where I have lived for some 35 years. Myriam Langford's apartment, number 1110, was located at the other end of the hall. The two of us progressively became the oldest tenants on the floor—oldest in age and in the length of time that we had been renting our apartments. The apartments situated between ours have for the most part been occupied for shorter periods, principally by younger persons enrolled as students in the medical, law, or business schools of the University of Pennsylvania, or at the Curtis Institute of Music.

In October 2014, although Myriam's health had begun to decline and she now needed a full-time home health aide to assist her, our paths still occasionally crossed in the hall. In early November I heard from members of The Wellington's staff that she was ill enough to be hospitalized. She died in the hospital on November 16.

On November 20 I found a handwritten note addressed to me that had been slipped under my apartment door. "Dear Renée Fox," it read:

> I am one of Myriam Langford's daughters (the one in Germany) and I am staying in Mother's apartment. Claudia [another daughter] told me yesterday that you were here, which made me very happy because I was trying to figure out how to find you. Mother was very fond of you and had spoken to me of you with great warmth and admiration. So, I wanted to let you know when and where the funeral is going to be in case you might want to be there […]. Thank you for giving Mother shared moments of warmth and neighborly friendship. I know that she took joy in her time with you.

"Thank you for your beautiful note," I replied:

> Your mother and I had a most unusual relationship—one that I cherished. We never did anything together that was conventionally

social—like going out to have a meal together in a restaurant. And curiously, we never even crossed the thresholds of each other's apartment (Due to mutual shyness? Or too much respect for each other's privacy?). But we had long, warm, enjoyable conversations in the hall stretching between our apartments, and sometimes in The Wellington lobby.

I felt great respect and affection for your mother. She was what I consider to be a "real lady"—a graceful and gracious woman, with a lively spirit, a sense of humor, a reservoir of courage—and with what I intuited was a fascinating life history, including a career in the theatre (that she only mentioned). I looked forward to every encounter with her (accompanied by her ever-present dog). She referred often to her daughters, with discretion, but with what I felt was great pride in you, pleasure in your company, as well as palpable love.

I will miss her greatly. And I will never be able to walk in the hall of the eleventh floor of The Wellington Apartments without thinking of her.

Soon after Myriam's death I did something that I never thought of doing while she was alive. I Googled her name on my computer to see if I could learn anything more about her. What I discovered was that she was 86 years old at the time of her death—exactly my age. She had, indeed, been an actress who had studied at the American Academy of Dramatic Arts and the Actor's Studio in New York. And in 1968, she had persuaded the entertainment committee of the American Women's Club in Brussels, Belgium, to produce William Inge's play *Picnic*, which she directed with a fellow actor, Charles Besterman. It was a hit, which gave her and Besterman the impetus to found the American Theatre Company (ATC) in Brussels, in 1969. According to its mission statement, the ATC is "a voluntary, non-profit organization, dedicated to the presentation of a variety of American plays covering a diversity of genres." It has not only survived but flourished over the course of the past 45 years, becoming "one of the pre-eminent amateur English-language theatre groups" in Belgium.[1] Since 1994 the ATC, along with the Comedy Club and the Irish Theatre Group, with whom the ATC has formed a cooperative association to support theatre, has been housed in a complex known as the Warehouse Studio Theatre, located in the Schaerbeek municipality of Brussels.[2]

These aspects of Myriam Langford's professional history coincided with events that occurred during a very significant interlude in my own professional life. Like her, I spent a great deal of time in Belgium during the 1960s, where

---

[1] "The American Theatre Company." http://www.atcbrussels.com/.
[2] "American Theatre Company (Brussels)." http://atc.theatreinbrussels.com/theatre/.

the sociological research I had launched on social and cultural factors that affected medical research and research careers in that country progressively evolved into a study of Belgian society "through the windows of its medical laboratories," and subsequently led me to the ex-Belgian Congo, where still another important phase of my life took place. Although during my Belgian years I did not move in the theatrical circles of which Myriam was a part, there was one deeply meaningful way in which I also became involved in the world of the theatre there. This was through the extraordinary friendship that I developed with the renowned Belgian dramatist, Michel de Ghelderode, and his wife, Jeanne. I frequently traveled to Schaerbeek—the district of Brussels where the ATC came to be located—to visit the de Ghelderodes, whose apartment was located there. In the salon of the Ghelderodes' apartment, which was as spellbindingly furnished as a brilliant stage set, Michel de Ghelderode, the master playwright, evocatively transported me into the "buried strangeness" of Belgium through the timbre of his voice, his dramatic gestures, and what he referred to as the "collection of imponderable objects" assembled around him.[3]

I am sorry that Myriam Langford and I never realized that among the things we shared was our past relationship to Brussels, Belgium, and the theatre in that setting. Knowing this would have enriched the conversations we carried on for many years in the hallway between our apartments, and increased the pleasure we had in them.

---

[3] I have written more extensively about de Ghelderode and my friendship with him and his wife in "Les Roses, Mademoiselle! The Universe of Michel de Ghelderode," a chapter in my book *In the Belgian Château: The Spirit and Culture of a European Society in an Age of Change* (Chicago: Ivan R. Dee, 1994), pp. 181–204. This chapter was reprinted in *The American Scholar* 63, no. 3 (Summer 1994): 403–19.

Chapter 4

MAKING AN APARTMENT
HOUSE MY HOME

In spring 2016 I received an unexpected message from Allan Domb, the real estate developer who owns The Wellington apartment house in which I live. "Dr. Renée Fox," he wrote:

> I just wanted to take a moment to personally thank you for making The Wellington your home for the past 37 years. It is the long-term residents such as yourself that truly make The Wellington a great place to live.
>
> All of the staff at The Wellington have nothing but fond memories of the interactions with you over the years.
>
> Please remember the staff is here for you at any time.

The Wellington, built in 1925 and renovated in 1987, is a 15-story building with 114 studio, one-, two- and three-bedroom rental apartments. A member of its staff vehemently expressed his conviction to me one day that the building should be called The Wellington *House*, rather than The Wellington Apartments, because, he said, "it is beyond just being an apartment building. It is the home of those who live here." It has certainly felt like *my* home for the almost four decades that I have inhabited apartment number 1103/4. For this I am indebted to the personnel of The Wellington—to how they view their jobs, and to the kind of relationship I have with them.

* * *

Greg, The Wellington's chief daytime front-deskman, and I estimate that 70 percent of the house's tenants are young women and men.[1] Many of them are studying for advanced business degrees at the Wharton School of the University of Pennsylvania. Others are physicians or nurses who work in

---

[1] All the names of the members of the Wellington staff in this essay are pseudonyms.

university-associated hospitals and who are in early postgraduate phases of their medical careers. Before the Curtis Institute of Music built a residence hall, a sizeable number of the school's students rented apartments in the house, among them a voice student who lived in an apartment adjacent to mine for a while and whose practice sessions were audible through our shared wall. Only rarely has a married couple with a baby or a small child lived here, although a number of the young single persons and married and unmarried couples have a cherished dog or cat. A much smaller group of The Wellington tenants are older retired persons. They have typically moved into Philadelphia's Center City from the suburban homes where they raised their children. They find urban living in the area where The Wellington is located—with its surrounding shops and restaurants, its institutions of art, music, science and education, and its historic landmarks—both attractive and conveniently accessible. They tend to be longer-term residents of The Wellington than the younger tenants, who are both literally and figuratively "moving on" with their lives.

* * *

The core staff of The Wellington is composed of 15 persons: 5 full-time, 5 part-time and 1 "fill-in" member of the front desk and front door staff; 2 persons responsible for maintenance; and 2 porters. All of them are African Americans—among whom one has Caribbean and another Liberian origins. Only one, a part-time member of the desk and door staff, is a woman. The house also has a property manager who is a white man.

The staff members belong to the Property Service Workers Union. Their shop steward is one of the front-deskmen. The door and desk personnel and the porters earn $16.27 an hour, and the two maintenance men $18.17 an hour. Although they are not compensated in higher wages for having worked more years at The Wellington, seniority is recognized with extra days of vacation. They all receive Blue Cross health insurance.

Several of the staff learned about the availability of the jobs they now hold through what appears to be a network of African American men who are employed by apartment houses in the Rittenhouse Square area where The Wellington is located, or by certain stores in the neighborhood—among them the deli-restaurant half a block away from The Wellington. One of the members of The Wellington staff told me with apparent pride that he remembers which takeout sandwich I recurrently ordered when he worked there.

Jobs held by staff members before they were employed at The Wellington also include: working as a doorman at another Rittenhouse Square apartment house; being employed by hospitality services in a hotel located in the square; stocking shelves in a chain store; serving as a security guard for a clothing store; acting as a salesman in a men's haberdashery; clerking in a state liquor store; being a jeweler for the first black jeweler in Philadelphia; assisting a hairdresser and cosmetologist in a beauty salon; being engaged as a mail carrier; working in a cleaning position in an Episcopalian church; loading airplanes for US Airways at the Philadelphia airport; and working for a hospital—in one case, as a technician in the Dietetics and Nutrition Department and in another, as a patient transporter in the Radiology Department. Two members of the staff served in the military before they came to work at The Wellington.

In addition to their jobs at The Wellington, several of the staff are involved in quasi-occupational extramural activities. Louis conducts some business in the field of numismatics, identifying and grading coins. Valerian, who "loves music," engages in occasional performances, as a drummer or a saxophonist. And Prudence is an amateur artist who privately paints and sculpts.

All the members of The Wellington staff attended high school—some with more enthusiasm and success than others. For Amal, school was a "challenge," and in a way it was also a "mystery." "My body was there, but not my mind," is the way he put it. He played basketball and baseball during his high school years—especially baseball, which is still his "passion." He has learned above all by observing and listening to people, he says. Greg was bussed into the high school he attended. Its student body at the time was predominantly white. He especially liked his English courses, loved to read, and was a member of the school's varsity football team. His father wanted him to go on to college, but this did not come to pass, partly because he did not receive the football scholarship he applied for. "I could have gone further," he once wistfully remarked to me, "and if I had, I was leaning towards studying criminal justice, and the possibility of becoming a probation officer." Louis, who completed two years of college, told me that he has as many as three licenses—as a beautician, a jeweler and a numismatist. And Valerian graduated from a business institute in New York City, where he studied computerized accounting.

Several staff members have children who are attending or who graduated from college. Amal showed me a photograph of his daughter clad in a cap and gown on the day of her college graduation. At the very moment when she received her diploma, he said, the sun came out, and he burst into tears.

When the staff speak about their families with me—which they often do—it is always with esteem for their grandparents as well as for their parents, and with gratitude for the roles the grandparents played in conveying to them "what the right things in life are": including being humble, having confidence, working hard and "doing good." Anton testified that although his maternal grandmother could not read or write, she emphasized to him the importance of having an education. Greg and Anton also give credit to how positively their values and behavior were influenced by the small rural communities in

Alabama and North Carolina, where they spent some of their years as boys and younger men. The staff express gratitude, too, for the help they have received from their spouses in keeping them "on a good track" and for the contributions made to the family's income and support by the jobs they hold. They are all full of praise for their children's accomplishments, particularly for their educational achievements; and they express pride in the number of grandchildren they have. Greg, who has eight grandchildren, carries in his wallet a photo of the one most recently born, which he was happy to show me.

Staff members also make mention of shadows and dark occurrences in their lives and the lives of some members of their families—including being apprehended by the police for incidents with a stolen car and with intoxicated aggression, having an uncle in jail, and being the parent of a son who has "constantly been in and out of trouble."

For several members of the staff their work and the relationships with colleagues and tenants that it involves has morally elevating significance. "It saved me from the horrors of the street that I saw growing up […] from the gangs and the guns," Amal contends. And Anton feels that it has improved his character, his "ability to render service," and his self-confidence. "I no longer go from job to job, as I used to," he testifies. "Once I got here, I decided this was the place I wanted to stay." "You never know who will give you the encouragement that you need to improve," he has remarked, and thanked me for being one of those people.

In a variety of ways, religion has an important place in the lives of most of the staff. Greg's grandmother was an evangelist, and he and his wife and children belong to an evangelically oriented Baptist church. From behind The Wellington's front desk where he is seated during his hours at work, he devoutly reads passages from the Bible twice a day. He is currently mentoring a young man in his church whom his grandmother "entrusted" to him. This role is giving him "great satisfaction," he told me, because his mentee is "doing well" in his daily life and is attending a community college.

Louis is a Muslim who is engaged in the activities of his local mosque. He is proud that he is sufficiently fluent in Arabic to read the original, untranslated text of the Koran, a copy of which he often brings to work. He seems especially to enjoy engaging me in conversations about religion. And whenever I have a visitor who is identifiable as a clergyman because he is wearing a clerical collar, Louis greets him with great respect and notable pleasure.

Trent, although not a regular churchgoer, once told me, "I learn a little from every religion." He is proud that he, and his grandmother before him, worked on the cleaning staff of an historic Episcopalian church in Philadelphia.

Prudence and her family have never belonged to any one church, but she says that she has had "a special relationship to God for a long time." There are numerous religious influences in her background, which were mediated primarily by her father, who reared the children. "His spirit is in each one of his children," she declares. Marcus Garvey, Father Divine, Judaism, the Bible and the Torah are among those religious influences, which she described as "a mixture of everything—a potpourri." What all these influences have in common, she attests, is "Truth"; that "there is something greater at work in the world than man"; that "we should do what we are supposed to do"; that we are extensions of one another"; and that "we receive in relationship to what we give."

I do not know what church Anton belongs to, but in my conversations with him he has referred to the bishop of his church in West Philadelphia from whom he receives good advice and who "thinks well of the man I have become." He has also told me that he sings in the choir of his church.

"I'm not religious," Amal contends, "but I'm generous, and I like to help others [...]. Service, caring for each other, and kindness under one roof" is what he calls his "legacy"—a legacy that has some relationship to the Gospels of Saint Paul and Saint Peter, and to his belief that it will be rewarded by God.

"I love people, and I love to keep people happy! It brings joy to my heart!!" Valerian, the deskman of Liberian origins has exuberantly declared to me. In this connection, he invoked an African, rather than a Christian saying that means "God will reward us for this," in recognition of the years that he knows I spent doing research in the Democratic Republic of Congo, and my abidingly deep identification with sub-Saharan Africa.

* * *

These are the people who help me navigate entering and exiting through the front door of The Wellington with my walker, and getting out of taxis and cars; who offer not only to go across the street to the La Colombe café to purchase a cappuccino decaf coffee for me, but even to accompany me if I want to take a short walk;[2] who respond immediately to whatever maintenance problems I encounter with plumbing, electricity, heat or air conditioning; who have come to my rescue a number of times when I have fallen in my apartment, and assisted me to get back on my feet; who continually engage me in lively conversation; and who greet my visitors with courteous warmth and interest. In these ways, and many others, they make me feel that they

---

[2] This offer has been made by Prudence, who has had experience working in a hospital and as a patient who was the recipient of a kidney transplant. She knows that I have done research and written about organ transplantation.

genuinely care about me, my well-being, and my ability to function—and, without invading my privacy, about how I live my life.

In The Wellington lobby, visitors are asked by a doorman or a desk person whom they have come to see and what their name is. Then their presence is announced by phone to the tenant on whom they are calling. Many of my visitors have told me how struck they are by the tone of voice in which Wellington staff members refer to me as "**DOCTOR** Fox"—as though, one of them said, "the title of 'Doctor' was written in bold, italicized, capital letters." I am treated with the extraordinary respect that their tone of voice implies; and although I have tried to convince staff members that they know me long enough and well enough not to address me with such deference, I have never succeeded in deterring them from doing so. "You earned it!" (the title of Doctor), a front-deskman succinctly replied to me once when I made this suggestion.

To my great embarrassment, I have also come to be seen as uncommonly intelligent by the staff. Louis informed me that he has told his mother about the "brilliance" of the conversations he and I have had; and the thank-you note that I received from Greg this past Christmas in response to my holiday gift to him began: "To one of the most brilliant women I have ever known." Contributing to their exaggerated assessment of my intellect and my professional status, and also to the ways in which the staff assists and supports me more than the job requires, are their esteem and affection for elderly people—including another Wellington tenant, a woman of some age several staff members have mentioned to me, whom they describe with admiration and enjoyment as "the feisty lady who lives on the sixteenth floor."

* * *

I have received two physical gifts from members of The Wellington staff. One is an ancient coin from Louis that is labeled on the sealed cardboard packet in which it is contained: "Biblical Coin 632 AD." The other is a large, multicolored ball fashioned by Valerian out of a countless number of rubber bands, on whose surface he has printed in black India ink: "To Dr. R. Fox. From Valerian." I keep the coin on the desk in my study and the ball on a counter in my kitchen, where I can continually see them. I cherish them above all because they are tangible, symbolic expressions of the gifts that I receive every day from The Wellington staff that transform what would otherwise be an impersonal apartment house building into my personal home.

Part 2

BEYOND BORDERS

Chapter 5

BEYOND BORDERS

How and why did it come to pass that my life as a sociologist has transported me far beyond the borders of my native land, of my origins and of myself?

I grew up in a socially homogeneous New York City neighborhood—a kind of "golden ghetto" on the Upper West Side of Manhattan. Its inhabitants were predominantly prosperous, nouveau riche, middle- and upper-middle-class Jewish families of second generation, East European ancestry, whose husbands or fathers were largely clothing business entrepreneurs. I knew virtually nothing about the lives my maternal and paternal grandparents had led in Russia and Romania, as they were reluctant to speak about their experiences before they migrated to the United States.

Despite the circumscribed nature of my childhood in these respects, I have memories that suggest that from an early age I was eager to learn about what life was like in other countries, and was encouraged by my parents to do so. One of the most vivid of these memories turns around the "Children of All Lands" series of books by Madeline Brandeis, which she dedicated "To every child in every land [...]. May you learn to love each other." I cherished *Little Jeanne of France*, one of the books in the series that my parents gave me, and they responded to my enthusiasm about this story of a little girl in France during and following World War I by giving me Brandeis's *Little Philippe of Belgium*, *Little Anne of Canada* and *Mitz and Fritz of Germany*.

The outbreak of World War II in Europe in 1939 and the subsequent Japanese attack on Pearl Harbor in 1941 shattered the long-standing isolationist tendencies of the United States. These world events also broke through the insularity of my home community with the arrival in the neighborhood of a sizable number of German and German-speaking Jewish families, who had the foresight and means to flee from the Holocaust genocide of some six million Jews by the Nazi regime in Germany and in German-occupied territories.

* * *

The years I spent in Harvard's Department of Social Relations from 1949 to 1954 studying for my PhD in sociology contributed in fundamental ways to the intellectual and moral importance I increasingly attached to social and cultural knowledge that transcended American society. To begin with, many of my male classmates were World War II veterans whose enrollment in graduate education had been made possible by the G.I. Bill.[1] They brought to their studies "an interest in learning more about the areas of the world in which they had fought and been posted, and the hopeful conviction that if knowledgeable understanding were extended beyond the boundaries of their own society to encompass other societies and cultures, the chances of a third world war might be diminished."[2]

Their presence and outlook contributed to the atmosphere and the ethos of the Department of Social Relations, whose faculty were in an effervescent phase of collaboratively constructing "'a common language for the social sciences,' and […] forging 'a general theory of action' that would apply to personality, cultural, and social systems" and their interrelationships.[3] Within that framework, irrespective of whether we were intending to become sociologists, anthropologists, or social or clinical psychologists, all graduate students were required to take the same introductory courses in sociology, anthropology and social and clinical psychology.

The anthropology course in particular expanded my cultural horizons as I came to appreciate more vividly the veracity of another underlying premise of the Social Relations Department—namely, how comparative knowledge of other societies could help one see more clearly the distinctive attributes of one's own society. In this course I read monographs by such illustrious anthropologists as Bronislaw Malinowski, Raymond Firth, E. E. Evans Pritchard and Margaret Mead, which carried me to communities in the Trobriand Islands, on the Polynesian island of Tikopia, in sub-Saharan Africa, in Samoa, and in Papua, New Guinea, where these scholars had conducted their field research.[4] These works also introduced me to the power of participant observation-based ethnography—the firsthand, analytic and interpretive method of social scientific inquiry that, in the words of anthropologist

---

[1] The G.I. Bill—the Servicemen's Readjustment Act—was signed into law in June 1944. It provided veteran beneficiaries with funds for tuition and books and contributed to their living expenses while they attended colleges and universities of their choice.

[2] Renée C. Fox, *In the Field*, p. 72.

[3] Ibid.

[4] Among the monographs I read were: *Argonauts of the Western Pacific*, by Bronislaw Malinowski (along with his volume of essays, *Magic, Science, and Religion*); *We, the Tikopia: A Sociological Study of Kinship in Primitive Polynesia*, by Raymond Firth; *The Nuer: A Description of the Modes of Livelihood and Political Institutions of a Nilotic People*, by E. E. Evans-Pritchard; and *Coming of Age in Samoa: A Psychological Study of Primitive Youth for Western Civilisation* and *Growing Up in New Guinea: A Comparative Study of Primitive Education*, by Margaret Mead.

Clifford Geertz, is also a "thickly descriptive" genre of writing with the evocative, "being there," capacity to take a person deeply inside another culture.[5]

My acquaintance with the research by two of the most groundbreakingly intelligent of my classmates through their doctoral dissertations conveyed me to still other places: to Java, where Clifford Geertz was conducting an anthropological field study of religious life in the town of Modjukuto; and to Japan, the site of Robert Bellah's sociological exploration of the historical roots of that country's modern economic development in its Buddhist, Confucian and Shinto religious traditions.[6]

Russia was another society my graduate studies introduced me to. In 1948, a year before I began my graduate work, Harvard established a Russian Research Center that was concerned with studying Russian institutions and behavior. One of its major intents was to further the understanding of the mainsprings of the Soviet Union and the Soviet world at a time when the Cold War was escalating, and to do so through fields of study that included sociology, psychology and anthropology. Two years later, in 1950, the so-called Harvard Project on the Soviet Social System was created within the center, under whose aegis extensive interviews were conducted with Soviet émigrés to West Germany, Austria and the United States. The project was developed by sociologist Alex Inkeles and social psychologist Raymond Bauer, who were faculty members in the Department of Social Relations. The two courses that I took with Inkeles on Soviet Russian society included material drawn from these interviews.

* * *

My PhD dissertation was based on the ethnographic study that I made over the course of 1951 through 1953 among the patients in an all-male, 15-bed, metabolic research ward in the Harvard Medical School–affiliated Peter Bent Brigham Hospital, and amid the 11 young Metabolic Group physicians who were both caring for these patients and conducting audacious, path-making research on them. The patients were seriously, often terminally, ill with medical conditions that at the time were not well understood scientifically and

---

[5] Clifford Geertz, "Thick Description: Toward an Interpretive Theory of Culture," in Clifford Geertz, *The Interpretation of Cultures* (New York: Basic Books, 1973), pp. 3–30. Clifford Geertz, "Being There: Anthropology and the Scene of Writing," in Clifford Geertz, *Works and Lives: The Anthropologist as Author* (Stanford, CA: Stanford University Press, 1988), pp. 1–24.

[6] Geertz's and Bellah's earliest published books grew out of their dissertations: Clifford Geertz, *The Religion of Java* (Chicago: University of Chicago Press, 1960), and Robert N. Bellah, *Tokugawa Religion: The Cultural Roots of Modern Japan* (New York: Free Press, 1957).

could not be effectively treated by established clinical means. Partly as a consequence of there being no effective medical treatment for their conditions, they had agreed to act as research subjects for the Metabolic Group. Although geographically speaking my study only required me to travel a few miles each day, from Cambridge, Massachusetts, where I lived, to Boston, where the hospital was located, my entry into the world of Ward F-Second and the Metabolic Group was akin—socially, culturally and psychologically—to arriving in a foreign land. Not only did I have to learn this world's medical language, I also had to come to understand the distinctive social system and culture of the tragicomic community that the patients and physicians had fashioned in response to the "experiment perilous" stresses and questions of meaning associated with the grave, inexorable illnesses, pain and suffering, medical uncertainty and therapeutic limitations, unintentional medical harm, risks of human experimentation and imminent deaths that they faced together.[7]

This study launched me on the six decades of ethnographic research in which I have engaged. My questing, pervaded by ethical and existential "experiment perilous" themes, has been centrally concerned with social and cultural aspects of health, illness and medicine; medical research (especially patient-oriented clinical research associated with organ transplantation, dialysis and the development and deployment of an artificial heart); the education and socialization of medical students and neophyte physicians; the significance and limitations of bioethics; and medical humanitarian action. It has involved "horizontal journeying" into deep layers of the lives and "way[s]-of-being-in-the world" of people in faraway as well as nearby places and, through them, "vertical journeying" into recesses of my own life in ways that have transcended the boundaries of myself, my society and my culture.[8]

* * *

[7] The phrase "experiment perilous" is taken from Hippocrates' aphorism "Life is short/ And the art long/The occasion instant/Experiment perilous/Decision difficult." It became the title of the book that grew out of my dissertation: Renée C. Fox, *Experiment Perilous: Physicians and Patients Facing the Unknown* (Glencoe, IL: Free Press, 1959; paperback ed., Philadelphia: University of Pennsylvania Press, 1974. Republished with a new epilogue by the author, New Brunswick, NJ: Transaction Publishers, 1997).

[8] Renée C. Fox, "Exploring the Moral and Spiritual Dimensions of Society and Medicine," in Carla M. Messikomer, Judith P. Swazey and Allen Glicksman, eds., *Essays in Honor of Renée C. Fox* (New Brunswick, NJ: Transaction Publishers, 2003), pp. 257–71, p. 266, and Renée C. Fox, "Observations and Reflections of a Perpetual Fieldworker," *Annals of the American Academy of Political and Social Science* 595 (September 2004): 309–26, 310. The phrase "a way of being-in-the-world" quoted in this article is one that I once heard the physician and anthropologist Arthur Kleinman use.

Over time my research moved progressively beyond the borders of the United States to European, African and Asian lands. My initial research trips to Europe were propelled by the relationships I had developed with young European physicians who were members of the Brigham's Metabolic Group. They had come to the United States soon after World War II to receive post-doctoral training that would prepare them for academic clinical research careers in their home countries. I became interested in why they were apprehensively unsure about whether they would be able to conduct this kind of research and pursue such careers in what they described as the "Old Europe" to which they would be returning. During the summer of 1959, supported by letters of introduction from Belgian, English, French and Swiss members of the Metabolic Group, and from the group's director, physician-in-chief of the Brigham,[9] I embarked on a European journey to explore what I pedantically phrased as "how social, cultural, and historical factors affected clinical medical research and medical research careers in contemporary Western European societies." My trip began in Belgium, from which I proceeded to visit London, Paris, Geneva and Zurich, where I conducted extensive interviews with junior and senior physicians and medical scientists in a number of university and research institute settings. When I returned to Belgium, I interviewed physicians and medical scientists associated with its four major universities (the universities of Brussels, Ghent, Liège and Louvain), the loci of most of the country's medical research. I was struck by how each of these universities embodied, in a semi-cloistered way, a particularistic cluster of Belgium's linguistic, religious, philosophical and political differences. That sociological observation was a paramount factor in the decision I made at the end of the summer that I would continue with the research I had undertaken, and that the core of my study would be situated in Belgium where, magnified by the country's smallness, a set of Western European institutional and cultural variables were intricately and intriguingly present. In a number of the articles and several of the books I have published, I have written in some detail about how through the ethnographic research that I conducted in Belgium over the course of many subsequent years, and the reactions of Belgians to it, my project evolved into what I came to think of as "Belgium through the windows of its medical laboratories."[10]

---

[9] This was Dr. George W. Thorn, the Hersey Professor of Medicine at Harvard Medical School.

[10] See Renée C. Fox, "An American Sociologist in the Land of Belgian Medical Research," in Philip E. Hammond, ed., *Sociologists at Work* (New York: Harper and Row, 1964), 345–91; Renée C. Fox, "Why Belgium?," *European Journal of Sociology* 19, no. 2 (1978): 811–16;

In turn, this enlarged, societal conception of my research in Belgium led to my first trip to the ex-Belgian Congo, in 1962, and to my ensuing decade of research there. One of its precipitants occurred on June 30, 1960, the day Belgium officially granted independence to the Congo, when I had the opportunity to observe firsthand how widely the loss of their African colony affected Belgians, and how emotionally they responded to it. It convinced me that having knowledge of the relationship between Belgium and the Congo, and comprehending the meaning that the Congo had for Belgians in more than political and economic ways, was crucial to my fully understanding Belgian society. But it is unlikely that I would ever have had the chance to become deeply involved in the Congo were it not for the entrance into my life at this juncture of Willy De Craemer, a Belgian sociologist who was a Jesuit priest, a missionary in the Congo, and the newly appointed director of the Centre de Recherches Sociologiques that had just been founded in Léopoldville by the episcopate of the Catholic Church in the Congo.[11] He recognized, and validated before anyone else, the kind of macro-knowledge of Belgium and insight into its society and culture that I had obtained through my medical research inquiry. He was impressed with what my ethnographic methods of research had yielded—including the implications that my observations and analysis might have for bringing about what he considered to be desirable social change. And he astutely predicted that because my findings challenged traditional, deeply entrenched societal patterns, they would evoke indignant as well as appreciative reactions in Belgian settings that extended beyond the sphere of medicine.[12]

In consultation with Father Victor Mertens, the Jesuit Provincial in Central Africa, and with Guy Mosmans, the White Father who was the general secretary of the episcopate of the Catholic Church in the Congo, Willy arranged for me to make a three-week trip to the Congo as a consultant.[13] The intent

---

Renée C. Fox, *In the Belgian Château: The Spirit and Culture of a European Society in an Age of Change* (Chicago: Ivan R. Dee, 1994); and Renée C. Fox, *In the Field*, esp. pp. 123–58.

[11] Léopoldville was renamed Kinshasa by Mobutu Sese Seko when he became president of the ex-Belgian Congo and renamed the entire country Zaïre. While the capital is still known as Kinshasa, the name of the country has been changed once more, to the République Démocratique du Congo.

[12] For an account of the circumstances surrounding my initial encounter with Willy De Craemer, of the relationship that developed between us, and also of his social background and the wellsprings of his calling to the priesthood, see Renée C. Fox, *In the Field*, pp. 146–49, and Renée C. Fox, "The House and the Family on Isegemsestraat," in *In the Belgian Château*, pp. 147–80.

[13] The White Fathers (*Pères Blancs*) are members of an international Catholic missionary society. Their name derives from the white cassocks they wear.

was for me to bring my sociological training, my experience in conducting social research, and certain aspects of my understanding of Belgium to bear on the plans that had been initiated for the development of the Centre de Recherches Sociologiques. The center was being inaugurated at a time when major change was taking place both within the Congo, during the first years of the country's independence from colonial rule, and in the Catholic Church, which was at that time addressing its relationship to the modern world in the sessions of the Second Vatican Council. The foundational premises of the center and its underlying goals were to produce firsthand "sociological research of scientific value" and publishable quality which would provide illuminating and useful knowledge and understanding of life in the Congo since independence. The center was especially dedicated to illuminating the challenges the country's culture, institutions and population were facing—information that would be of interest not only to Catholic clergy and laypersons in the Congo but also to an international, "ecumenical" readership that extended beyond the country and the church.[14]

At the end of this initial visit to the Congo, I was invited to become the center's scientific advisor and its American liaison—appointments that I unhesitatingly accepted. Over the course of the next five years, under the direction of Willy De Craemer with the collaboration of a small staff of two Congolese colleagues, a Belgian *Scheutist* priest and two Spanish women and one German woman who were members of lay religious Catholic organizations, the center undertook numerous wide-ranging research projects in different arenas and areas of the country which I helped to design and in which I participated. The projects involved a broad spectrum of quantitative and qualitative methods of inquiry, all of which required going directly into the field. Notable studies were of the occupational and social aspirations of the country's secondary school students; of the Congo's medical assistants and the emergence of the country's first African physicians from among them; of several of the religious movements that abounded on the Congolese scene; of the everyday realities of Congolese family life, including the painful conditions to

---

[14] Another seminal figure in the founding and orientation of the Centre de Recherches Sociologiques was Joseph Von Wing, a then elderly and retired pioneer Jesuit missionary in the Lower Congo and a renowned ethnographer of the Kongo tribe who had been an advisor to the Colonial Council in Brussels in the former Belgian Congo. One of the characteristics that he, Mosmans, and De Craemer shared was that each of them, before the Congo's independence, had pressured the Belgian colonial administration to provide greater opportunities for Congolese to obtain an advanced education and to accord them more responsibility for managing the affairs of the country. Their shared perspective on colonialism and its injustices was an important latent influence in the creation of the center and in its outlook.

which many women were subject; and even of the Congo Rebellion of 1964–1965, which entailed physically following its trail as it spread from one region of the country to another.[15]

I look back with wonder on my years in the Congo, especially when I contemplate the number of factors that converged to transport and deeply involve me there. They included my experience in conducting ethnographic research and the trained capacity it afforded me to move from micro to macro levels of analysis which the metamorphosis of my research in Belgium entailed; the historical time when this research took place; how it was viewed and acted upon by those who inaugurated and animated the Centre de Recherches Sociologiques; my readiness to go where my research carried me; my espousal of the social as well as the intellectual goals of the center; and also the support of my parents, who gave me their encouraging approval for this venture and even provided me with a first-class Brussels/Léopoldville/Brussels Sabena airline ticket for my initial trip to the Congo.

To this day, however, I continue to feel that these contributing factors do not thoroughly explain how and why it came to pass that I was accorded the responsibility and trust that I received from members of the Catholic clergy in the Congo—including from those of ecclesiastical rank and authority. For, after all, as I wrote in my autobiography, when I first appeared on the Congolese scene I was "a relatively young person in her early thirties, […] an unmarried laywoman, of American nationality, with only junior, assistant professor status in academia," devoid of any prior experience in Central Africa "who, rather than being a Catholic, or even a Christian, was Jewish, and whose life ordinarily unfolded in a secular world." On these grounds, I could have been considered dubiously qualified, "an outsider, and as an unattached young woman, […] someone to be kept at a politely measured distance from

---

[15] For a more detailed account of the persons I met, the places I visited, the discussions in which I engaged, and the observations I made during these weeks in the Congo, see Fox, *In the Field*, pp. 159–74. For a fuller list of the research projects that the Center undertook, see Fox, *In the Field*, pp. 177–78. Among the publications that resulted from this research were: Willy De Craemer and Renée C. Fox, *The Emerging Physician: A Sociological Approach to the Development of a Congolese Medical Profession*, Hoover Institution on War, Revolution and Peace, Stanford University, *Hoover Institution Studies* 19 (1968); Willy De Craemer, *The Jamaa and the Church: A Bantu Catholic Movement in Zaïre*, Oxford Studies in African Affairs (Oxford: Oxford University Press, 1977); Renée C. Fox, Wily De Craemer and Jean-Marie Ribeaucort, "'The Second Independence': A Case Study of the Kwilu Rebellion in the Congo," *Comparative Studies in Society and History* 8, no. 1 (October 1976): 78–109; Willy De Craemer, Jan Vansina and Renée C. Fox, "Religious Movements in Central Africa," *Comparative Studies in Society and History* 18, no. 4 (October 1978): 458–75; and Willy De Craemer, "A Cross-Cultural Perspective on Personhood," *Health and Society* (*Milbank Memorial Fund Quarterly*) 61, no. 1 (Winter 1983): 19–34.

the celibate, masculine communities of consecrated priests." Instead, in the words of Father Mosmans, through the process of spiritual "discernment" in which priests like him were trained to engage, they seemed to regard my having been "pointed […] towards Africa and the Congo" as "truly providential."[16] When I look back on what led me to the Congo, and what happened when I got there, and consider the significance it still has for me, I cannot blithely dismiss his interpretation of how and why it came to pass.

* * *

The years of research that I conducted in Belgium and the Congo were not done at the expense of my teaching as a faculty member in the sociology department at Barnard College. With the exception of the one sabbatical year that I spent in the field, this research was conducted during long academic summers and Christmas/New Year vacations. I thought of myself primarily as a teacher and secondarily as a researcher, and I had great pleasure in teaching, and in the relationships that I developed with students. Nevertheless, a major tension existed between my teaching and research—namely, the limited extent to which I had a chance to integrate the content of what I was learning through my research into the courses I taught. This situation existed primarily because the faculty of Barnard's sociology department consisted of only four members; because I was the junior member among them, even after I was promoted to a tenured associate professorship; and because, as a consequence of my junior status, I was perennially expected to teach certain of the required courses for sociology majors—particularly Introductory Sociology and Methods of Social Research. Teaching the required courses curtailed my opportunity to develop new courses to an extent that hindered my chance even to introduce a course in the sociology of medicine—my area of special interest and competence—into the curriculum. What was more, my colleagues did not seem to attach much pedagogical value to what I might be able to convey to students by incorporating more cross-cultural material and an enlarged international perspective into my teaching.

Primarily for these reasons, without acrimony and with gratitude for all that had been happily meaningful about my 11 years as a Barnard faculty member, I decided that the time had come to leave the college and seek another position. I was supported in this decision by trusted persons from whom I sought counsel, including my foremost teacher and mentor, the renowned sociologist Talcott Parsons, who acknowledged that my research in Belgium and the Congo had carried me to "new intellectual places" and that my situation at

---

[16] Fox, *In the Field*, pp. 170–71.

Barnard was "restricted." I realized that leaving Barnard was risky, especially because at that time I was one of the few women sociologists in the United States who occupied a tenured position in academia, and there was no guarantee that I would be able to obtain another. But I was willing to take that risk because of the importance to me of what was at stake.

* * *

The circumstances surrounding my three successive journeys to the People's Republic of China (PRC) over the course of 1978 to 1985, and the research that I undertook there, differed greatly from those associated with my research in Belgium and the Congo. It was the historic November 14 to December 3, 1978, trip to China by the Board of the American Association for the Advancement of Science (AAAS), of which I was a member, that inaugurated this interlude in my professional life.[17] At that time, the American government was on the threshold of "normalizing" its relationship to the PRC. Normalization officially took place on December 16, when a "Joint Communiqué on the Establishment of Diplomatic Relations between the United States of America and the People's Republic of China" was issued, after which, on January 1, 1979, the two countries formally established embassies in each other's capital. It was in this context that AAAS was given the "unofficially official" anticipatory role of taking steps toward opening up bilateral scientific and technological cooperation and exchanges between the United States and the PRC. The mission of the AAAS board's 1978 trip was to explore and informally begin to develop this kind of collaboration. The concrete arrangements for the trip were made by the China Association for Science and Technology (CAST), which has described itself as "the largest national non-governmental organization of scientific and technological workers in China" which "also serves as the bridge that links the Communist Party of China and the Chinese government to the country's science and technology community."[18] Members of CAST's national and local staff accompanied us wherever we went. Our itinerary began in Beijing, and from there we traveled to Shanghai, Guillin and Canton, visiting many scientific and educational institutions and giving public lectures in some of these settings on topics about which we had previously informed the Chinese Liaison Office in Washington, DC, we were prepared to speak. Just before we left Beijing, at our audience in the Great

---

[17] For a more detailed ethnographic account of my first trip to China, see Renée C. Fox, *In the Field*, pp. 273–98.

[18] This description of the China Association for Science and Technology at one time appeared in Wikipedia.

Hall of the People with Vice Premier Fang Yi, who was then China's top government official in the sphere of science and technology, we received his oral mandate to foster scientific collaboration between CAST and AAAS through the contacts with Chinese scientists that we were about to have.

It became apparent that our Chinese interlocutors were far more familiar with the physical and biological sciences than with the social sciences, and more responsive to them; that none of them had ever heard of medical sociology, my field of expertise; and that they were unacquainted with the participant observation-based way in which I conducted research. I was therefore very surprised three years later, in 1981, when I received an invitation from CAST, transmitted via AAAS, to revisit China in order to introduce the subject of medical sociology and my mode of social research to a number of Chinese medical settings. The person who was chiefly responsible for this invitation was Mr. Yu Qiyu, the deputy chief of the Division of the Americas and Oceania of the Department of International Affairs of CAST, a poet and scholar whose knowledge extended far beyond science and technology to include European and American as well as classical Chinese literature, and European philosophy in addition to Confucianism and Marxist thought. As an emissary of CAST, in the course of a number of trips he made to the United States during 1979 and 1981, he paid several visits to me in Philadelphia and engaged me in deep conversation about medical sociology and my relationship to it, during which it became apparent that he had thoughtfully read some of my publications. He expressed appreciation for the fact that they involved "going into reality [...] in natural settings" rather than the "emptiness" of purely abstract thinking; that they recognized the human qualities and the "social community" connections of the "living beings" who peopled them; that they also dealt with moral issues; and, as he eloquently expressed it, that, like "Chinese window pictures," the micro-studies I had made opened onto "larger landscapes."

Through negotiations with William Carey, the executive officer of AAAS, it was agreed that I would spend six weeks in China in the summer of 1981 accompanied by the medical historian Judith Swazey—an especially close colleague, coresearcher, coauthor and friend—and that the details of our itinerary and program would be entrusted to Mr. Yu. The primary site that he selected and arranged for our field research was the First Central Hospital in Tianjin, a major city and seaport in northern China. It was a sociologically brilliant choice. The prominent urban hospital that Mr. Yu had found for us contained within its walls many of the phenomena and issues on which Judith and I had previously focused our research and writing, including the treatment of critical medical conditions (in the only free-standing intensive care unit in China); the deployment of hemodialysis for kidney failure; exploratory steps toward undertaking organ transplantation; leadership in nursing education; and strongly committed involvement in developing what the hospital termed a system and process of "medical morality" to deal with "shortcomings" and "mistakes" in the delivery of medical and nursing care.[19]

The fascinating and fruitful time we spent in this setting was deemed to be "very successful" by Mr. Yu, who closely followed our research, visited us while we were in Tianjin, and read our subsequent publications about it. "You [...] achieved [...] some real heart to heart communication in Tianjin," he wrote to me much later:

> Your observation [...] was very sensitive [...]. Your field study spirit, taking fact finding and empirical study as [a] basis, [...] allowed you to get to the root, to the truth below the surface. I believe your deep understanding of the real situation in Tianjin First People's Hospital served as a microscope for you to perceive the whole picture over China [...]. During a time after about thirty years of isolation, Chinese intellectuals had limited knowledge about either [...] medical science or medical sociology in the West.

Mr. Yu also acted as the intermediary for my third journey to China—this time "solo"—during the summer of 1985, when I conducted field research at the Yangpu District Tumor Hospital in Shanghai, spent time as an observer in the laboratory of an immunologist engaged in research relevant to liver cancer in another Shanghai hospital, and made a trip back to the Tianjin First Central Hospital to see how the situation there had developed since 1981.

* * *

My relationship with Mr. Yu continued through correspondence and through my publications that I sent him, at his request, until his death from prostate cancer in 2014. Enclosed inside the elaborately beautiful greeting card printed in Chinese and English that I received from him every Christmas and New Year season was a long letter from him, penned in his exquisite, calligraphy-like handwriting. One of his last such messages to me contained his comments on the book about Doctors Without Borders which I had recently published:

---

[19] For details about our experiences in Tianjin see Fox, *In the Field*, pp. 299–318, and Renée C. Fox and Judith P. Swazey, "Medical Morality Is Not Bioethics: Medical Ethics in China and the United States," *Perspectives in Biology and Medicine* 27, no. 4 (Spring 1984): 336–60.

Your significant chronicle record helps greatly to make [this] humanitarian effort known to many people who had been blind to [it], [...]
including myself [...]. It activated in my mind an old maxim in China
deeply buried in my memory. It reads: The better the care that you give
to the aged and young kids of other families, the more secure will be the
life of the aged and young kids in your own family [...]. May a united
worldwide effort be able to serve all people in a way that is a promotion
of China's old maxim.

Mr. Yu not only played a crucial part in organizing the arrangements for the
times that I spent in China. He also indispensably contributed to the acceptance
and cooperation that I received in the field there, and to the "understanding
of the real situation" in the settings I observed and their "Chinese-ness" which
he generously said I had achieved.

"No account of fieldwork would be complete without acknowledgment of
the pivotal role that informants play in the conduct of ethnographic research,"
I have written:

> There is a sense in which virtually all the members of a group, an organ-
> ization, a community or a population being studied in this way take
> part in the research. But there are certain individuals among them with
> whom the fieldworker develops a particularly close and collegial rela-
> tionship. In effect, this special kind of informant becomes the partici-
> pant observer's observing participant, adviser, and counselor and, in
> many instances, more than a friend.[20]

Mr. Yu was such a "companion in the field." In my research in China, in
Belgium, and in the Congo, in the many milieus of Doctors Without Borders,
and also in the hospital world of Ward F-Second, it was persons like him who
played cardinal roles in making it possible for me to move beyond my own
social, cultural and personal borders. I am profoundly grateful and indebted
to them for that.

* * *

Of all the field research that I have undertaken, it is my study of the medical humanitarian organization Doctors Without Borders/Médecins Sans
Frontières (MSF) whose duration in time, and whose geographical, societal

---

[20] Renée C. Fox, "Observations and Reflections of a Perpetual Fieldworker," 309–26,
324–25.

and cultural scope, have been the greatest. It began in 1993, grew out of my research in Belgium, France and the Democratic Republic of Congo, continued for more than twenty years, and carried me to numerous Western European countries, Russia and South Africa. The travel this questing has involved, and the time I devoted to it, are associated with my convictions about the value of living my life in a way that is not confined to the place where I happen to have been born, or to the social "boxes" of my origins. Deeper than this is the importance I attach to human interconnectedness, empathy and solidarity; and to being vitally in touch, on a worldwide scale, with the experiences and problems of others—including and especially with those that entail suffering and injustice. For this reason, I have found great personal as well as socio-logical meaning in learning about the principles and value commitments of Doctors Without Borders through my in-the-field ethnographic research; observing how they implement their principles and values in the missions they undertake; and tuning in on the "culture of debate" way in which they self-critically examine their precepts, decisions and actions. That meaning was eloquently expressed in a statement about the essences of MSF that I heard during a lecture Sophie Delaunay gave while she was making a transition to a new position in the organization. She had been an active member of MSF for 22 years, serving in multiple capacities in a myriad of countries:

> I don't know what MSF will be tomorrow. But I do know its strengths and its weaknesses. Both are the reasons why I love this organization and its members dearly.
>
> I hope I was able to convey the sense that for me and my colleagues assistance goes far beyond the simple programmatic delivery of medical care. Care is first about caring about others as if they were oneself, or those we love. Care is about taking the risk of rejecting the status quo when it seems unacceptable. MSF is one among many actors in the field of humanitarian action. And each of us plays a specific role. We don't claim to be the ministry of health of the world. We don't claim to restore peace. We feel okay about just keeping alive and healthy as many indi-viduals as possible every year, and about showing a face of humanity and solidarity to communities when their world falls apart [...]. Each contribution to humanitarian crises is as valuable as the other, as long as we don't claim to be what we are not.[21]

* * *

---

[21] Sophie Delaunay, "Saving the World, or Saving One Life at a Time? Lessons My Career with Médecins Sans Frontières (MSF) Has Taught Me," the Seventh Annual Renée

I hope that without falsely or pretentiously claiming "to be what I am not," or exaggerating what I have accomplished, I have been able to transmit such a sense of "humanity and solidarity" through the in-the-field and beyond-borders nature of the sociological research in which I have engaged, and its relationship to my writing and my teaching.

C. Fox Lecture in Medicine, Culture and Society, delivered at Medical Grounds Rounds, Department of Medicine, University of Pennsylvania Perelman School of Medicine, in the Flyers/76ers Surgery Theatre, on May 5, 2015.

Chapter 6

THE MEANINGS OF MY MSF BOOK

Doctors Without Borders: Humanitarian Quests, Impossible Dreams of Médecins Sans Frontières was published in the spring of 2014. Like my other books published over the sixty years of my professional career, *Doctors Without Borders* is a work of medical sociology based primarily on ethnographic field research and written in a narrative style. It has much in common with its antecedents, although it differs from them in ways that are connected with the special meanings the book has for me.

My relationship to the medical humanitarian organization MSF (the acronym for Médecins Sans Frontières, its French—and original—name) is a long-standing one and continues to this day. My initial contact with MSF took place in its Brussels and Paris offices in the early 1990s, at a time when I was in the midst of other sociological research in Belgium, France, and the Democratic Republic of Congo. From the outset I was drawn by "the values that MSF espoused, and that its members concretized through their medical humanitarian action," and these values significantly influenced my decision to embark on a firsthand study of MSF. As I have written, the organization's "principles in action coincided with some of my own most basic and strongly felt values." It was my hope that the research I was undertaking would bring me closer to the relationship of disease and sickness to poverty, inequality and social injustice—which I considered to be "the most critical social and moral issues associated with health, illness, and medicine." I also hoped to better understand the human suffering associated with, and action to ameliorate, these issues, in part because "more than occasionally in the past, I had found myself questioning whether the topics to which I had devoted so much of my research and writing [had been] too remotely connected with these issues, and too detached from action to ameliorate them."[1]

---

[1] See Renée C. Fox, "Exploring the Moral and Spiritual Dimensions of Society and Medicine," in Carla Messikomer, Judith P. Swazey and Allen Glicksman, eds., *Society and Medicine: Essays in Honor of Renée C. Fox* (New Brunswick, NJ: Transaction Publishers, 2003), pp. 257–71, p. 268; Renée C. Fox, *In the Field*, p. 367; Renée C. Fox, *Doctors Without*

Over the many years of research that ensued, MSF Belgium and MSF France, two of the organization's most important operational sections, remained my primary launching pads for trips to observe its members in action in the field. I also visited the national offices of many of MSF's other 17 sections. I attended the organization's periodic international meetings and conducted intensive field research in Athens, Cape Town and Moscow. In all these contexts I was given unconditional access to illuminating primary and secondary documents. And I was continually in contact with a number of MSF's many websites. The welcoming openness and collaborative willingness with which members of MSF responded to me and to my research activities emanated from their shared commitment to principles of transparency and accountability, from the coincidence of their commitment to being in the field in proximity to the people they assisted and my in situ field methods of research, and from their collective conviction that "ideas matter for action."

The physical presence that my research entailed, its interactive nature, the extensive geographical area that it covered and the exceptionally prolonged time over which it took place, gradually transformed my status among MSF members into what one of them termed an "insider-outsider." I increasingly experienced my name being recognized among MSFers, and those I interviewed, and with whom I corresponded, intimated that they thought I was becoming very knowledgeable about MSF and was acquiring an unusual degree of understanding of their culture as well. In this latter regard, in keeping with MSF's collective penchant for self-examination and self-criticism, and what I eventually came to call their "culture of debate," it appeared to be especially important to them that I seemed to be taking note of some of their shortcomings, perplexities, dilemmas and conflicts, while also chronicling their aspirations and achievements. An ongoing email correspondence developed between certain MSF members and me, and I had occasional conversations with some of them via Skype. Among the correspondents there were those who attested to the value they felt of looking back at some of their MSF experiences—particularly the challenging and troubling ones— "through your eyes," as one of them put it. I also received visits from MSFers whose travels brought them close enough to my apartment in Philadelphia for them to feel it was feasible to stop by. One such visitor took photographs of the files that contain all my MSF field notes and documents, which are located in what I call the "Archives" room of my apartment. I was both amused and

---

Borders: Humanitarian Quests, Impossible Dreams of Médecins Sans Frontières (Baltimore: Johns Hopkins University Press, 2014), pp. 2–3.

intrigued by this incident. It made me wonder whether one of the ways in which I had come to be viewed was as a valued keeper of MSF's ongoing history and its memories.

* * *

My attendance at MSF's 40th anniversary meeting, which took place in December 16–18, 2011, in Saint-Denis (a commune on the outskirts of Paris with many immigrant inhabitants and a high unemployment rate), constituted the last interlude of field research that I conducted inside the organization. By this time I was in the midst of writing the *Doctors Without Borders* book—an endeavor that had begun towards the end of 2010. For the finale of the book I planned an ethnographic account of that anniversary meeting and a meta-analysis of its implications. (This account became the book's "Remembering the Past and Envisioning the Future" coda.)

The all-consuming process of writing the book continued steadily, with remarkably little stress, throughout 2012. In January 2013, I entrusted the manuscript to Jack Beatty, a professional editor, who judged it to need relatively light editing, which we collaboratively completed in the course of March. Meanwhile, through the intermediary of the professor of medicine and medical history, Kenneth Ludmerer, I submitted the table of contents and several sample chapters to Johns Hopkins University Press, hoping that they would be interested in publishing it. The press's Faculty Editorial Board promptly reviewed those materials and, on April 17, approved an "advance contract." Six days later the press received the entire manuscript from me. After obtaining outside reviews, the board definitively accepted the book on July 17, 2013. Exactly one year from the approval of the contract, in mid-April 2014, printed copies of the book arrived at the press's warehouse. And on June 1, 2014, the book made its official publication and marketing debut.

The swiftness with which the writing and publishing of the book occurred is notable. But looked at from another point of view, taking into account the years of research from which the book grew, I was 65 years old when I made my first contacts with MSF and 85 years old when my book about it was published. What is even more remarkable than the years involved in research and writing is that throughout all those years my interlocutors in MSF continued to express a lively interest in the book I intended to write, and none of them ever asked me why it was taking so long. Quite the contrary. Immediately after the book's publication, I received an email message from one of the members of MSF who had known me the longest.

He wrote:

> This book would never have come to completion if it were not for the resilience and immense personal contribution at the personal cost of its author, who managed to overcome numerous logistical and administrative barriers to be a direct witness of key MSF events during the last 20 years. […] At a time when everything needs to be expedited—fast delivered at the cost of being superficial—you undertook this mammoth task of observing MSF for the last 20 years, and you completed this daunting marathon.

What touched me the most about this message was that I felt it contained an implicit tribute to what its sender believed had been my ability to fulfill some of MSF's own important values.

Furthermore, MSF members never gave me the impression that they considered me to be old, and getting progressively older, in ways that would adversely affect the quality of my research or the book that would eventually emerge from it. Rather, even when I reached my mid-80s, they continued to treat me as a respected and knowledgeable elder whose professional history and experience in doing firsthand research in a number of different MSF milieus had a certain kindredship with their own frontline, international action in the field.

Writing this paragraph calls to mind what I considered to be the most moving event that took place at MSF's 40th anniversary meeting: the interlude when three of the physicians—all of them men in their 70s—who were among the founders of MSF described with passion some of their lived experiences in the early years of the organization's existence.[2] At the conclusion of their presentations they received a prolonged standing ovation from the entire audience which seemed to me to express the great respect that this relatively young, exceptionally vigorous, action-oriented assemblage had for persons of age, as well as their gratitude for the role that these physicians had played in MSF's history.

* * *

The process of publishing the MSF book brought me into an unexpectedly close relationship with the Books Division staff of Johns Hopkins University Press. From the outset, my book was deeply understood as well as appreciated by them—especially by the press's executive editor Jacqueline ("Jackie")

---

[2] Fox, *Doctors Without Borders*, pp. 257–60.

Wehmueller, who shepherded the book and me through the phased movements toward publication, and with whom a mutual personal friendship developed. The praise that I once received from her for "manag[ing] to infuse [the book] with joy and humor, despite the sadness and misery of the stories it tells," was of great importance to me because of its relationship to a view of the world and of the human condition within it that I feel members of MSF and I share.

An indicator of how responsive the Hopkins press staff was to the book and its author is the poster they presented to me when the book was published. At its center is a miniature version of the front jacket of the book with its title, author's name, and photograph of the Khayelitsha township in Cape Town, South Africa, the site of a major MSF HIV/AIDS program. Below it is written, in handsome script, *"With gratitude."* It is signed by 23 members of the Acquisitions, Manuscript Editing, Design and Production, and Marketing departments of the Books Division.

The reactions of members of MSF to the published book were encouragingly positive. The MSF-USA New York office posted a notice about the book's publication on its website. "You describe and capture MSF better than we could ever do," a member wrote to me. Another testified that "the rigor of scholars like you, and the passion" help to "unravel [...] the complexity" of what is happening in MSF and the societies in which it is working. One member asked me to sign an extra copy of the book for her daughter to read when she grew up—a copy that was hand delivered to her by an MSF colleague from the United States, when they were both attending an international meeting in Amsterdam. The MSF office in Berlin arranged a Skype session with me to discuss the book and my experiences with MSF. Dubbing themselves "Renée's Berlin Book Club," those who participated sent me a cosigned note after the session, thanking me for "the new insights about our work that we all received," pledging to "keep reading," and inviting me to meet with them again. And one of the most senior, long-term members of MSF made the prediction that the book would "become a reference in the MSF world," which he portrayed as "condemned to be amnesiac [through its] lack of organized institutional memory." He thanked me "for helping the young generation [in MSF] to understand where we come from and be better informed in drawing future lines of a movement [...] to which I have given most of my professional life."

Sophie Delaunay, who was then executive director of MSF-USA, reviewed *Doctors Without Borders* for the journal *Perspectives in Biology and Medicine*, describing the book as "a refreshing and unusual perspective on this larger-than-life organization": "With the candor and attention to detail a social scientist can marshal, Fox takes us backstage where MSFers breathe, agonize, exult, or fulminate to defend a complex and imperfect idea of humanitarian action." "Fox examines how MSF generates and processes internal crises and finally rises from the ashes," she wrote, adding:

> Reading through the chosen field studies reversed my original skepticism and made me feel grateful to the author for not focusing on more pre-dictable flagship missions. Both case studies are extremely informative about how MSF decided whether to act and about what it considers a medical humanitarian basis for action. And both illustrate the long, pol-itically sensitive process of getting national and international decision-makers to adopt and implement better health policies. In the end, even for someone who has been affiliated with MSF for two decades, these stories gave me an almost jubilant sense of uncovering original food for thought.[3]

The only negatively critical comment about the book that I received from MSF sources came from someone who said that what I had written about MSF was "too kind." I was delighted with this remark, because it was con-sistent with what I portrayed in the book as MSF's "anti-heroic heroism" and its self-critical "culture of debate."

Illustrating that culture of debate for MSF for many years was Samuel Hanryon, a member of the Communications Department of MSF France who uses "Brax" as his nom de plume. Brax's brilliant cartoons illustrate my book, too—depicting gender roles, the limits of humanitarian action, the global nature of MSF, the difficulty of reaching a consensus among MSF's various sections and members, and the broader, "Impossible Dream," goal of conquering illness worldwide. In my ongoing correspondence with one MSF member I recently learned that during an international MSF general assembly in Johannesburg which provided a "key moment for reflections on where MSF is," the assembled members learned the "sad news" that Brax had decided to leave MSF to join the International Federation of Human Rights. My corres-pondent noted: "I mentioned to everyone I could, including Joanne Liu, our inspiring international president, your analysis of MSF: 'an equilibrium mir-acle' with such a large size and with so little hierarchy, probably helped a great deal by someone like Brax who regularly managed to turn political crises into a big laughing exercise.'" Now that Brax has left, my correspondent wrote, "I am anxious about future MSF acrimonious debates." Not at all accidental is that Brax's last cartoon for MSF depicted comically grotesque, physically vio-lent confrontations among MSF staffers. In French and English some of them

---

[3] Sophie Delaunay, *Perspectives in Biology and Medicine* 59, no. 3 (Summer 2016): 437–44, p. 439.

call out, "Do we agree to publicly disagree?" and others respond, "Yes! We agree!" Printed so inconspicuously in very small letters in the bottom left-hand corner of the cartoon that it could easily be missed are the words "BYE BYE BRAX"—his farewell message. The self-mocking imagery of the cartoon and of its captions are both quintessentially Brax and quintessentially MSF.

* * *

My book appeared during the early months of the outbreak of Ebola in Guinea, Liberia and Sierra Leone. At that time, MSF was one of the only humanitarian organizations on the ground in these West African countries, caring for those afflicted with this deadly hemorrhagic viral disease, attempting to curtail its spread, and signaling to the world at large that the unprecedented epidemic proportions it had assumed in these settings called for a massive intervention on the part of the international community. The vital treatment, contact tracing and surveillance roles that MSF was playing in responding to the epidemic, and the prescient witnessing and advocacy in which they were engaged in calling the gravity of the epidemic to the world's attention, evoked widespread public interest in and admiration for MSF. As a consequence, my newly published book received more notice from the media than it otherwise would have. I was interviewed by journalists from *The New York Times* and *Bloomberg News*. An extensive online interview with me was carried by the *Daily History.org* website. Dan Rodricks, a columnist for the *Baltimore Sun* and the host of a talk show on WYPR FM, Baltimore's public radio station, conducted an hour-long broadcast interview with me. And, accompanied by a cameraman, Fred de Sam Lazaro, a distinguished correspondent with PBS, the national American public television network, traveled to my apartment in Philadelphia to interview me for a Religion and Ethics Newsweekly program about MSF that also was telecast on a PBS Friday Night *NewsHour*.

* * *

Five years after the publication of my book, MSF's members continue to keep me informed about important meetings, and about the major issues that are discussed at these meetings. They provide me with copies of some of their documents that are still in draft, as well as those that have been issued. They share personal and family news with me:

Our children dispersed around the world: our son now with MSF in Kunduz, Afghanistan, trying to re-construct a symbol of nonpartisan humanitarian medical help, replacing the US-bombed hospital, while war is bitterer than ever between occupation forces and Taliban's. Our daughter is coming close to finishing her sixth year of medical school [in Australia] and already registered to do all her elective here in SA, in a former mission hospital in Eastern Cape as well as in one of Cape Town referral hospital to learn about infectious disease.

And they even write to me in undaunted detail about field missions in which they are deeply immersed:

MSF needed an interim Head of Mission in Juba, South Sudan, so here I am. [...] I don't know how they are going to get things sorted here. There is such a crazy system of patronage that people have bought into, and humanitarian workers no longer have real respect or protection. [...] This is such a different context to what I had in 2005–2010 where we could really expand medical care. Let's also add the start of a Kala Azar outbreak. [...] I have to say, I'm very glad to come in and lend a hand.

The hospital itself is impressive. It's still primarily a tented camp. The first prefabricated container walls have come in for a few units, but our next delivery truck is stuck in a swamp somewhere between Bentiu and Juba. [...]

The first two tents shelter the malnourished kids. There are 14 beds in each tent. A lot of the children are accompanied by a mother and a grandmother, and sometimes 2 or 3 siblings who could not be left at home. We're always watching out that they don't become sick while hanging out with us.

The next 4 tents are for the sick kids—here we have up to 20 little ones per tent. Last month it was a lot of malaria and this week it looks like pneumonia is on the rise. Many of the oxygen concentrators have double tubes so the kids can share. The most amazing thing is seeing their progress from being either unresponsive or crying in abject pain in Tent 1, and then as they wind their way through to Tent 4 just before discharge.

Right next door are the adult patient tents—recovering gunshot wounds, abscesses, severe malaria and those few cases we are still trying to diagnose.

Maternity has a couple of modular container units—makes it a little easier to care for the mothers who are about to deliver and those just recovering alongside premature babies. There were even three sets of twins when I was there the day before yesterday.

I have also had very meaningful and enjoyable meetings with MSF members in academic settings. During a two-day visit to Yale University as a guest lecturer in April 2015, I was invited by Unni Karunakara, previously an international president of MSF who was then a visiting fellow at Yale, to teach with him a session of his seminar on humanitarian action. The seminar took place in a conference room around a table on which a pad, a ballpoint pen and a green apple had been set out for each of the student-participants. At the close of the class, Unni stood up and placed one green apple on the top of my head, another on the top of his own, and, while holding both of them in place, asked a colleague who was attending the seminar to take a picture of us with her cell phone. What might have impelled Unni's act, I speculated, was an association with the tale of William Tell, the legendary hero of Swiss independence and freedom, who when ordered by a tyrannical Austrian ruler to shoot an apple off the top of his son's head with an arrow from his crossbow, succeeded in doing so without injuring his son; or perhaps, I thought, Unni connected it with the aphorism, "An apple for the teacher." But when I asked him about it, he told me that what he had had in mind was *The Son of Man*, the self-portrait painted by René Magritte that depicts a man in an overcoat and a bowler hat, whose face is obscured by a green apple that hovers in front of it. "Magritte was a Belgian artist, and you spent many years doing research in Belgium," Unni explained, and "in addition, you have the same first name—René(e)." When I look at the framed photograph of the two of us standing side by side with apples on our heads that now occupies a prominent place in my study, I marvel at Unni's erudite quick-wittedness. I delight in the self-mocking Doctors Without Borders' genre of humor that his gesture with the apples expressed. I also feel gratitude for the symbolic way in which he recognized my research in Belgium, and how it led to my study of Doctors Without Borders.

Two weeks later I had the opportunity to spend time with Sophie Delaunay, who in May 2015 came to the University of Pennsylvania School of Medicine from MSF's New York office to give the seventh annual Renée C. Fox Lecture in Medicine, Culture and Society. Although we had not met face-to-face previously, we had come to know each other through my research inside of MSF and a warm email correspondence. I had proposed her to the members of the selection committee for the Fox Lecture as a candidate to give this endowed lecture. Sophie was amenable to my suggestion that she center her talk on her 22 years of experience as a humanitarian worker with MSF. "Saving the World, or Saving One Life at a Time? Lessons My Career with Médecins Sans Frontières Has Taught Me" was the title she chose for it. Everyone in the filled auditorium was moved by her testimony about what it was like for her and her colleagues in MSF to be trying to "alleviate suffering on this earth" through the "imperfect offering" of the care they give—the joys and the sorrows it involves, the achievements and failures, and the human tragedy and human comedy. They were also impressed by the eloquence, authenticity and lack of egoism with which she delivered her message. And I was profoundly honored not only by her acceptance of the invitation to give this lecture but by the reference she made to me in her introductory remarks. "Renée is well known in MSF for all the work she's done in analyzing the ethos and the culture of our organization—and the many contradictions within it," she told the audience. "We in MSF, and myself personally," she went on to say, have "respect and admiration" for what she characterized as my "sharp, non-complacent, ethical and humanistic reading of [their] complex work."

* * *

My chronicle of the ways in which this book and the years of research behind it enduringly connect me with MSF, its reason for being, and its members would be incomplete without mention of a beautiful bouquet of lilies that I received this spring. They were hand-delivered to me in my apartment by a member of the Berlin section of MSF who was spending several days in Philadelphia. She had been charged by the director of the Berlin office to pay me a visit while she was here, and to bring me the flowers with her greetings. What is more, she took photos of me to show to her colleagues upon her return to Berlin.

Chapter 7

VENTURING OUT WITH
A ROLLING WALKER

My muscles are now too weak, my posture both too rigid and too bent, and my balance too precarious for me to walk without some means of support. And so, I move about with the assistance of a walker—a so-called rollator that is sometimes referred to as a "wheeled walker."[1] Mine has a bright blue metal frame; four wheels; two handlebars with hand breaks that can be lifted upward, to slow the walker's movement, and downward, to halt it completely; and a black padded seat and black wire shopping basket. These are standard attributes of a rollator. But my walker has an additional feature. Perched on its handlebars is a squeezable bicycle horn in the shape of an "extraterrestrial alien" with a pea green small body and a large head and big, dark blue, pupilless eyes. The alien is seated, with its tiny hands wrapped around its knees. It was purchased for me by my physical therapist, who thought that when I was making my way down a crowded street, sounding that horn would be an amusingly effective way to signal to passersby that I was approaching.[2]

Managing my walker inside my apartment is a blandly routine everyday affair. It is only when I leave my apartment and move into public spaces that I experience the social encounters and the physical challenges that using a walker can entail.

---

[1] The rollator was invented in the late 1970s by Aina Wifalk, a Swedish woman who contracted polio in 1949 at the age of 21, when she was training as a nurse. Although the physical handicaps she was left with as a consequence of polio forced her to give up plans for a nursing career, she went on to become a disability counselor. Her years of professional experience in this role, and her personal experience of walking with long, underarm crutches that took a toll on her body, led her to conceive of a new kind of walking aid on wheels. See "Walker(mobility)," *Wikipedia*, en.wikipedia.org/wiki/Walker_(mobility); "Aina Wifalk," *Wikipedia*, http://translate.google.com/translate?hl=en&sl=sv&u=https://sv.wikipedia.org/wiki/Aina_Wifalk&prev=search.

[2] The walker featured in the cover photograph is the one I began using several months after this chapter was written.

My neighborhood is an upscale urban area, well tended by the city and by the apartment and commercial buildings, the businesses and the stores located within it. Nevertheless, it confronts a pedestrian wheeling a walker along its streets with numerous physical hazards. To begin with, there are all the bumps and cracks in the pavement to watch out for, the metal grates and covered manholes to circumvent and the small pools of water in the gutters (seeping out of imperfectly drained sewers) that it would be best to leap over, if I could—especially during winter months when they freeze. There are also the many nonautomatic doors to stores and restaurants that take strength to open, and those that threaten my balance because they must be pulled rather than pushed open. Paradoxically, most challenging are the curb cuts that the city is legislatively required to install at intersections to help people with disabilities cross the street. The majority of these ramp-like cuts are sloped so steeply that a walker or a wheelchair could roll out of a person's control when moving down them, and someone on crutches or using a cane could pitch forward and fall.

A person using a walker must be vigilantly aware of human hazards in the streets. Foremost are the pedestrians whose self-preoccupation renders them oblivious to others. The most dangerous are individuals who are reading emails or texting on their cell phone as they walk. One of the more extreme examples of threatening incidents occurred when a young man who was talking on a cell phone and wearing ear plugs that insulated him from all sounds other than the voice of the person with whom he was conversing, and who was accompanied by a dog on a long leash in which I could have become entangled, almost collided with me. Then there are those who out of awkwardness, confusion or assertiveness try to push past me. I suppose that I should sound the "alien" bicycle horn atop my walker when such encounters occur, but I am deterred from honking by timidity, embarrassment about potentially attracting public attention and concern that startling such persons may cause them to move in ways that would further endanger me.

Dealing with the mothers and nannies pushing baby carriages who abound in my neighborhood is another matter. Partly because they are primarily focused on the interests of the children in their care, many of them seem to assume that they have the right-of-way when they approach curb cuts. Both because I, too, think they should have priority and because of my self-protective instincts, when we are approaching the same curb cut, I usually let them charge ahead of me before I tackle going up or down. As they pass by, many of the tots in carriages pique my sociological curiosity, because they stare at me and my walker with what seems to be fascination. I wish there were some way of knowing what intrigues them. Is it because I have a rolling vehicle that is like and also unlike their stroller?

I do not feel vulnerable to predators or wrongdoers as I move about. Quite to the contrary, I am impressed by the "kindness of strangers"[3] —by the many people, unknown to me, who reach out to help me move about. They make way for me on the street, assist me in getting around impediments, open doors for me, let me enter or exit from an elevator before they do, offer me their places on waiting lines. And they boost my morale as I pass them in the street by smiling at me in a friendly way, or greeting me with a "Hello," "Good morning," or "Have a good day."

Some individuals extend their aid in exceptional ways. I vividly remember, for instance, a young father wheeling a baby in a carriage and accompanied by a small boy on foot and a pet dog in tow, who nonetheless offered to help me go down a curb cut, and somehow managed to do so.[4] I have been impressed as well by the gentlemanly way in which burly construction workers and garbage collectors have gone out of their way to remove obstacles from my path—including moving their parked trucks so I can get by. One day when I was walking with unaccustomed nimbleness and speed down the street, the driver of a local garbage truck whom I often encounter called out to me in a friendly, humorous tone of voice that encouraged and empowered me: "Hi! Slow down! If you don't, I won't be able to catch up with you!"

But whatever their ages or occupations may be, it is African American women and men who most frequently—and with notable skill, respect and personal warmth—have lent me a hand. In the course of the conversations I have had with them, many have made reference to what their mothers had taught them about helping others and, some of them, to the fact that they were currently caring for their elderly mothers at home. When I have commented appreciatively on their adroitness in assisting me, some have told me that they have had training and experience working in a hospital or a nursing home. And there are those among them whose religious devoutness I have felt when, upon taking leave of me, they have said not only "Goodbye" but also "God bless you."

* * *

---

[3] "I have always depended on the kindness of strangers" is a line from Tennessee Williams's play *A Streetcar Named Desire*.

[4] It is sociologically interesting to me to notice that at present there are more fathers wheeling baby carriages on the street than there were in the past. Many of these fathers are accompanied by their wives who are walking alongside of them; some are not. The young father who helped me get down the curb was handling the carriage, the baby in it, his small son and the dog by himself.

The apogee of all my experiences traversing the streets with my walker came one afternoon when I was approaching an animated group of African American high school boys who spanned the breadth of the sidewalk. Before I had a chance even to consider how I could move around them, with unanimity and choreographic grace, they opened their ranks and made a pathway for me. Passing through their midst in this way made me feel as close as I ever will to having the Red Sea part, as recounted in the book of Exodus, and crossing safely over it to the dry land on the other side. I cannot imagine any happening related to navigating with my walker that will ever surpass this one. It did not surprise me. But it did deeply move me.

Chapter 8

ELECTION TO THE EXPLORERS CLUB

In a letter dated January 31, 2014, I received word that the Explorers Club's Board of Directors had approved my application for "membership as a Fellow National" of the Club. "Congratulations," the letter declared. "You are now part of our extraordinary family of Explorers, which was established over 110 years ago. As you know, you are part of a multidisciplinary, professional society dedicated to the advancement of field research, scientific exploration, resource conservation, and the ideal that it is vital to preserve the instinct to explore." The letter, signed by Alan H. Nichols, JD, DS, president of the Explorers Club, concluded with a statement of welcome to the club and the affirmation that "We look forward to sharing with you 'the spirit of exploration.'"

I had never heard of the Explorers Club until Dr. Mabel Purkerson strongly urged me to apply to be admitted to its membership. She offered to be my sponsor and to obtain the cosponsor who was required. She explained that because the club regarded itself as a fellowship-based community, sponsorship by two members of the club was an important component of the application process.

Dr. Purkerson, a professor emerita of Medicine at the Washington University School of Medicine, a pediatrician and a nephrologist renowned for her pioneering research on the pathophysiology of the kidney, is a prominent figure in the Explorers Club. She is the long-standing chair of its St. Louis Chapter and, at the national level, a member of the club's nominating, membership, Legacy Society, and archives and artifacts committees. In 2010 she was awarded the Sweeney Medal for her dedication and service to the club. The club's online biographical sketch of Dr. Purkerson describes her as having "a lifelong interest in nature, wildlife conservation and preservation"; "a wide experience in world travel [that] has enabled her to learn about other civilizations and observe people living in places visited—particularly those with environmental needs"; and "deep concern that our Planet's untamed beauty be preserved for future generations."

I was gratified by Dr. Purkerson's offer to support my application for membership in the club but surprised that she considered me qualified to be admitted to it as a fellow—a category defined in the club's application form as going "beyond the basic requirements of [a] Member to include […] contributions to scientific knowledge in the field of geographical exploration or allied sciences […] usually evidenced by scientific publications documenting fieldwork or explorations." Contributions to geographical exploration? How did this apply to me, I wondered?

The more information I sought and acquired about the club, the more it seemed to me that I was not just a dubious candidate, but a potential misfit. The club's mission, I learned, was: "To inspire exploration and protection of wild places from our backwoods to our oceans, mountain peaks and distant galaxies—while sustaining a spirit of fellowship among all explorers." Since its founding in 1904 the club has grown to include 26 chapters whose approximately three thousand members come from more than sixty countries and every continent on the globe. The members include leaders in aerospace exploration, archeology, astronomy, conservation, mountaineering, diving, ecology, geology, paleontology, physics, polar exploration, speleology and zoology. Club members were among the first to reach the North and South Poles, to summit the peak of Mount Everest, to dive to the deepest point in the world's oceans, to set foot on the Moon, and to pilot a solar-powered flight across the United States. A club member is a finalist for the Mars One mission to establish a human colony on Mars.[1]

* * *

I thought it inconceivable—in certain respects even absurd—to suppose that I was an appropriate candidate to be associated with the exploits of such famed and daring explorers. I was about to celebrate my 86th birthday, and it had become necessary for me to use a walker to navigate. I was hardly in a physical condition to scale mountains, plunge to the depths of seas, travel to the coldest places on Earth, or soar into space! And I have always had a distant, rather apprehensive relationship to the world of nature, the outdoors and animals—in effect, to the physical places and the forms of life to which Explorers Club members are boldly drawn and especially dedicated.

I was born and grew up in New York City, and I have lived and worked in cities all of my life. In many ways I am an urban creature as well as an urban

---

[1] See "Join the Club," https://explorers.org/about/join/join_the_club, and page 16 of *Explorers Club Inc. v. Diageo PLC*, sequence no. 001, index no. 152524/2014, Supreme Court of the State of New York County, part 53.

dweller—most familiar and at ease with city streets, buildings, neighborhoods, and apartments. When I was a child, during the school year, the closest I came to any contact with "nature" was to be taken on adult-chaperoned visits to the playgrounds in Riverside Park and Central Park, and to see the animals in the Central Park Zoo.

The possibility of having a family pet—a dog or a cat—was never even considered by my parents, and my mother's fear of dogs, which she attributed to having once been threateningly jumped on by a large German Shepherd, was transmitted to me. In the course of my lifetime I have developed an anxiety-free relationship with only two dogs. The dogs in question, Cognac and Molly, belonged to my close friend and colleague Judith Swazey, in whose home I have been a frequent, family-like guest. Both were dachshunds who, as Judith pointed out, were small enough for me to feel comfortable with. In the unique case of Molly, my fear was completely dispelled by the fact that— perhaps because she observed me moving about the house with the aid of a walker—her canine intuition led her to watch protectively over me.

Every summer my parents made arrangements to send me out of the city to a sleep-away summer camp in what they called "the country," in Upper New York State. Although I appreciated the scenic beauty of the lake at which the camp was situated, and of the mountains surrounding it, my fear of deep water greatly inhibited my swimming and canoeing capacities. Furthermore, with the possible exception of archery I did not have demonstrable athletic abilities in any land-based sports. Lodged as we were in solidly built wooden bunks, being a camper gave me no experience in pitching or living in a tent. And the campfires around which we gathered for certain ceremonial events were built and tended by our camp counselors.

My continuing fear of deep water curtailed the exercises that I did in a pool during the long and intensive rehabilitation process I underwent after contracting a severe case of poliomyelitis at the age of 17. It even threatened my graduation from college, until I summoned up enough determination to pass the swimming test that Smith College required.

When standing on the shoreline of an ocean, contemplating its depth and its vastness, the power of its waves, and the eternalness of its tides, or traveling through the boundless space and the vicissitudes of the sky as a passenger in an airplane, I have always experienced a frisson of existential angst—an acute sense of my smallness, my vulnerability and frailty, and my ultimate mortality.

On what conceivable basis, then, could I be accepted into the company of members of the Explorers Club like the polar explorers Roald Amundsen, Richard Byrd, and Robert Peary, mountaineers like Edmund Hillary, aviators like Charles Lindbergh and Chuck Yeager, astronauts like John Glenn, Buzz Aldrin, Neil Armstrong, and Sally Ride, or the primatologist-ethologist-anthropologist Jane Goodall, who conducted 45 years of firsthand research among chimpanzees in Tanzania, studying their social and family life?

* * *

In the end, it was Dr. Purkerson's enthusiasm about my applying for membership in the club that emboldened me to do so. The key part of the application form was its "exploration résumé" section, in which the applicant was asked to summarize his or her "expedition and research field work experiences, both vocational and avocational," and was encouraged to "add extra pages as required" to present his or her "accomplishments and contributions to exploration." Rather to my surprise, I did need extra pages.

I began my response by making reference to the titles and subtitles of two of my published books: *In the Field: A Sociologist's Journey* and *Doctors Without Borders: Humanitarian Quests and Impossible Dreams of Médecins Sans Frontières*. "The allusions to 'being in the field,' and to 'journeying' and 'questing' through sociological research," I continued "are not only metaphorical":

They characterize the quintessence of my life as a sociologist. Central to my career

has been the first-hand, participant observation–based, ethnographic field research that I have conducted, principally in the sociology of medicine [...]. The chief empirical foci of my studies have concerned phenomena associated with medical research and therapeutic innovation (especially related to hemodialysis, organ transplantation and artificial hearts); medical and medical professional education and socialization; medical humanitarian action; and bioethics. Over the course of more than sixty years, I have not only conducted such research in many American (US) milieus, but also through recurrent field trips of long duration in Western Europe (predominantly in Belgium and France, and in England, Switzerland and Greece as well); in Russia (Moscow and St. Petersburg); in Africa (especially the Democratic Republic of Congo—formerly Zaïre, and before that, the Belgian Congo) and South Africa (particularly Cape Town); and in the People's Republic of China (Beijing, Tianjin, and Shanghai) [...].

Almost all the books and articles that I have published over the span of my career (which are listed on pages 15–26 on my CV) are based on this research [...].

In my role as teacher [I concluded], I have shared what I have learned "in the field" through the courses I have given—including field methods of social research; and I have directed the dissertations of countless PhD students that were based on field research.

To my great surprise and gratification, the contents of my résumé were considered to be sufficient to admit me to membership in the club.

* * *

The numerous benefits the club accords to its members include subscriptions to its quarterly *Explorers Journal* and *Explorers Log*, its *Club Roster*, and its events newsletter; invitations to its annual Lowell Thomas dinner, public lectures, and exploration seminars; participation in events hosted by any of its 26 "worldwide" chapters; the chance to "network with fellow members for future expeditions"; and "the opportunity and honor [...] to carry the Explorers Club Flag on approved field expeditions." It is not imaginable that I will ever embark on such historic, flag-bearing expeditions. Nor is it even likely that I will be able to attend Explorer Club events that take place outside of Philadelphia, where I reside. But through the medium of the club's publications and website, I have been able to envision and vicariously participate in a wide range of its activities, such as when carrying Explorers Club Flag 206 with them, oceanographer and filmmaker Fabian Cousteau (grandson of Jacques Cousteau) and his team emerged from their 31-day mission of living underwater to study, document, and communicate the impact of pollution and climate change on the reefs of the Florida Keys.

Explorers Club publications and communications have also given me insight into the attitudes and values that its officers and members consider to be "pillars" of exploring and discovering—attitudes and values that are consonant with some of my own, even though I have not explored oceans, mountains, or space, as so many club members have:

> Mike Allsop presents a talk about inspiring others to live extraordinary lives, based on a philosophy that says if you truly believe you can accomplish something, then you will. Mike combines a career as a commercial airline pilot with an ongoing series of challenging adventures and expeditions. [...] His most recent exploit was running the world's highest-ever marathon that started at 18,000 ft. at the top of Kalapatar, which is next to Everest, crossing over the Cho Lo pass. The adventure has been turned into a film aimed at helping young people between the ages of 12 and 15 overcome fear of failure [...].

> Every one of Mike's adventures incorporates an element of giving back to others. This includes returning the famous Pangeboche Yeti skull

and hand to restore an income for a Nepalese monastery, to delivering tools and clothes to remote communities. Mike's February 2013 feat of running 7 marathons in 7 days on 7 continents raised over $75,000 for a New Zealand children's charity.[2]

* * *

Explorers have a reputation [...] of being "full of themselves." Some believe that a big ego is the road to big discoveries in the field. *I-centeredness* is not the same as *determination*, admittedly a factor in all major exploration finds. [...]

To the extent *I-centeredness* is, or borders on, selfishness, bragging, egotism and the like, it is likely to do more harm than good—certainly on an expedition involving other people [...]. We know it's easy to detect the member of the exploration team whose only interest is to be personally famous or rich or to get credit for the discovery.

Exploration is always a team activity, and anyone who ignores this will bear an extra burden to be successful.[3]

* * *

Among the many compelling Explorers Club communications I have received since my election, it is the report of the keynote address that was given via telecast at the club's 110th annual dinner by Stephen Hawking, one of the world's most brilliant theoretical physicists and cosmologists, that has had the most powerful meaning for me. Hawking is almost entirely paralyzed by a motor neuron disease related to amyotrophic lateral sclerosis (ALS) that confines him to a motorized wheelchair. He can communicate only by using a handheld pressure sensor, a speech-generating device to pick out words from an on-screen computer menu. And yet, through the genius of his intellect, his union of the general theory of relativity, quantum mechanics, and quantum gravity, and the buoyancy of his spirit, he has explored not only the vastness of our universe but also the possible existence of an infinity of other self-generating universes. Furthermore, with the exception of Australia, he has physically travelled to every continent on the globe—including to Antarctica. And he

---

[2] NYC—Lecture Series feat. Mike Allsop. https://explorers.org/events/detail/nyc_lecture_series_feat_mike_allsop.

[3] Alan Nichols, "On the Ascent," *Explorers Log* 46, no. 1 (Winter 2014): 1–2.

has gone under the sea in a submarine, up in a hot-air balloon, and on a zero-gravity flight in a specially modified plane. In addition, he has made it known that he is "booked to go into space with Virgin Galactic," the commercial spaceflight company planning suborbital space flights for tourists, science missions and launches of small satellites.[4]

"Not to leave planet Earth would be like castaways on a desert island not trying to escape," Hawking said in his address to the Explorers Club. "Sending humans to other planets [...] will shape the future of the human race in ways we don't yet understand, and may determine whether we have any future at all."[5]

It need hardly be said that I am not endowed with Hawking's awesome intelligence, cosmological vision or audacious courage. Even the thought of contemplating such phenomena as the beginning and the end of time, and such questions as "What is it that breathes fire into equations and makes a universe for them to describe?"[6] which he ebulliently tackles, frightens me. But I suppose it could be said that for a sociologist, I have traveled widely and quested broadly—at least within the confines of this planet.

I agree with Hawking that "handicapped people should concentrate on things that their handicap doesn't prevent them from doing and not regret those they can't do." And like him, I feel that I "have managed to do most things I wanted," and hope that I have added something to knowledge and understanding in the process.[7]

I wonder, though, whether Stephen Hawking has ever experienced anything like my unfettered dreaming space. I have been told that I sing, as well as talk out loud, when I am asleep. And quite mysteriously, in my dreams, I am never using a walker, a crutch or a cane. Only when I awake do I realize that in the realm to which I voyaged during my sleeping hours, I do not need them.

***

Stephen Hawking died in his home in Cambridge, England, on March 14, 2018, at the age of 76. As his funeral cortege arrived at Cambridge University's church, Great St. Mary's, its bell ran out 76 times—one for each year of his

---

[4] Stephen Hawking, *My Brief History* (New York: Bantam Books, 2013), p. 125.

[5] As reported by Megan Gannon in "Stephen Hawking Urges Explorers to Visit Other Planets," *Scientific American,* March 18, 2014. https://www.scientificamerican.com/article/stephen-hawking-urges-explorers-to-visit-other-planets/.

[6] A statement made by Hawking quoted in M. Mitchell Waldrop, "The Quantum Wave Function of the Universe," *Science* 242 (December 2, 1988): 1248–50, p. 1250.

[7] Hawking, *My Brief History*, pp. 122–23 and 126.

life. The vehicle was met with applause from the hundreds of persons who had gathered outside the church. As many as 500 persons attended the private service that was held for him. The choir of the Cambridge College, Gonville and Caius, where he had been a fellow for more than fifty years, performed a choral work—"Beyond the Night Sky"—which had been composed as a gift to him for his 75th birthday party.[8]

Two months later, on June 15, 2018, a service of thanksgiving was held for him at Westminster Abbey. His ashes were interred in the Nave of the Cathedral, near the graves of Sir Isaac Newton and Charles Darwin. The inscription on his slate stone is an English translation of a phrase that appears in Latin on Newton's gravestone:

HERE LIES WHAT WAS MORTAL OF
STEPHEN HAWKING 1942–2018

"The stone depicts a series of rings, surrounding a darker central ellipse. The ten characters of Hawking's equation express his idea that black holes in the universe are not entirely black but emit a glow, that would become known as Hawking radiation."[9]

---

[8] "Prof Stephen Hawking Funeral: Legacy 'Will Live Forever.'" BBC News. www.bbc.com/news/uk-england-cambridgeshire-43582950.

[9] "Stephen Hawking, Physicist, Scientist and Writer." www.westminster-abbey.org/abbey-commemorations/commemorations/stephen-hawking.

Part 3

MEDICAL ENCOUNTERS

Chapter 9

ENCOUNTERS WITH PHYSICIANS

I am fortunate that at my advanced age I do not have any serious illnesses. Even so, my calendar is filled with doctors' appointments. In the last few months I made office visits to my primary care physician, my eye doctor, my dentist and an oral surgeon. I also visited a hospital outpatient department for a bone mineral density scan that my primary care physician had ordered. Appointments with my gynecologist and my podiatrist are imminent.

I am mindful of how privileged I am to receive continual comprehensive care, and I am grateful for its benefits. But this care produces side effects that augment my awareness of the many ways in which my body and my psyche are beset with symptoms of aging—including multiple sorts and sites of discomfort, pain and paresthesia, reduced mobility, greater fragility, increased fatigue and elevated psychological and existential anxiety. My primary care physician candidly and humorously diagnosed this array of symptoms by reminding me that I *was 88 years old.*

* * *

It was the morning of my routine biannual checkup with Dr. Lilly, my primary care physician.[1] Her nurse assistant checked my medications list and took my blood pressure (which was heightened by the so-called white coat anxiety I experience at the outset of any medical visit), and then Dr. Lilly entered the examination room accompanied by a young man whom she introduced as a first-year medical student. He was spending the day with her, she explained, observing what the daily round of her practice was like. She asked my permission to allow him to sit in on my visit with her, which I readily granted. My consent and the positive sentiments that underlay it were associated with my career-long commitment to the role of a teacher, the gratifying experience I have had in teaching many premedical and medical students, and the years I have spent conducting empirical research on the educational and

---

[1] Physicians' names in this essay are pseudonyms.

socialization processes involved in becoming a physician. I anticipated that this student's presence would enhance the pleasure and meaningfulness the session with Dr. Lilly would have for me. But, contrary to my expectations, it turned out to be one of the most uncomfortable and disquieting interludes I have spent in her office.

To begin with, the slender, dark-haired, bespectacled student seemed to be huddled inside himself as well as inside the short, rumpled white coat he wore. He remained silent throughout the visit, neither asking a question nor making a comment. I had bought with me a handwritten short list of topics that I wanted to discuss with Dr. Lilly, or at least mention to her. These included symptoms of gastric reflux and constipation, the development of a sore on my lower gum and my growing reluctance to walk unaccompanied outside my apartment, even with the aid of my rolling walker, because of the problems of balance and navigation caused by the increasing torsion of my neck and scoliosis of my spine. As I reported these matters to her, I glanced intermittently at the student, whose inwardly turned cryptic expression I could not decipher. To my dismay, I unexpectedly found myself becoming increasingly concerned about the impression he might be forming of me on the basis of these medical "complaints." I felt as though this man more than 60 years younger than me, who had not yet developed the professional detachment that results from clinical training and experience, was being given access to overly intimate knowledge about my aging body.

Probably, partly in response to the reference I had made to my difficulties in walking independently outside of my apartment, Dr. Lilly informed the student that I had contracted a severe case of poliomyelitis in my youth, and that some of my current difficulties were "post-polio" concomitants. Seizing upon what I regarded as a conversational opportunity, I proceeded to share with him some details about the serious case of polio with which I had been afflicted. In retrospect, I realize that what impelled me to do this was my assumption not only that he would consider this information to be medically "interesting" but that it was the kind of information that might confer more dignity as well as seriousness on his view of me as a patient and a person.

Would I have felt less embarrassed and self-consciously elderly in the company of this student if he had been a communicative young woman rather than a taciturn young man; if he was far enough along in the medical school curriculum to have had more clinical experience; and if I had met him in an impersonal hospital setting rather than in my physician's office, where his presence intruded on the usual privacy of my one-on-one relationship to her? I think so.

In the course of my next appointment with Dr. Lilly I asked her to tell me a little more about the student who had been present during my previous visit, and I shared with her the ambivalence I had felt about that experience. On the one hand, I said, in keeping with the importance that I attach to medical education and my motivation to contribute to it, I was pleased that he was there. But somewhat to my surprise, I told her, I had also felt self-conscious and embarrassed to have him listening to the elderly woman I have become discussing the state of my digestion and bowels. Dr. Lilly's response was unexpected. Rather than talking with me about *my* reactions to the student, she proceeded to tell me about *hers*. She had been gratified by the enthusiasm he had expressed about the time he had spent inside a primary care practice, she told me, and he had asked her if he could come again—an opportunity that she had granted him in the form of two more day-long visits. With notable pleasure, she went on to say that he had heightened her awareness of some of the ways in which her practice was "really interesting."

"Why do you think your physician responded as she did?" a close friend asked me. That's an interesting question. Seeing her practice through the fresh eyes of a neophyte medical student, I speculated, seems to have raised her morale by at least temporarily dispelling what she ordinarily must have felt was routinely everyday about the primary care she is engaged in delivering. My friend did not find this explanation of Dr. Lilly's avoidance of my reaction to the student's presence fully satisfying.

* * *

Dr. Lilly believed that the time had come for me to have another bone mineral density scan (DEXA scan), because four years had passed since my last one. This scan is a form of x-ray technology used to measure bone mineral density and bone loss. It is performed on the lower spine and hips and is used most often to diagnose osteoporosis and to track the effects of treatment for this condition. Osteoporosis (a term derived from the Greek word for porous bones) is an age-related disorder causing the gradual loss of bone density and strength. It is more common in women, especially postmenopausal women, than in men. The chief dangers associated with it are the increased risk of bone fractures and their consequences.

My scan was performed in the Women's Imaging Center of the Radiology Department at Pennsylvania Hospital, where I was described in their medical records as an "88-year-old female, post menopause, [with] osteoporosis, a history of estrogen deficiency, on calcium therapy," and with "no specified reason for [the] exam." I knew that the scan would involve lying on my back, on a flat x-ray table, as a large scanning arm moved slowly over my body, while a narrow beam of x-rays passed through the part of my body being examined. A description of the procedure that I found on the internet reassuringly described it as quick, painless and safe, using "a much lower level of radiation than standard x-ray examinations"—so low, in fact, that the radiographer could stay in the room with the patient during the scan.[2]

There was every reason to expect the scan to be a routine, innocuous process. But for reasons that had nothing to do with the amount of radiation that was used or the discomfort of lying very still in a number of uncomfortable positions on a hard x-ray table, the scan unexpectedly turned out to be simultaneously stressful and perilous for me.

Before the scan, the radiographer needed to measure my weight and height. To provide this information I was required to step on to the unsteady platform of the medical scale in the scan room, and to stand as erectly as I could so the rod attached to the scale could be used to measure my height. That I need a walker to navigate, that without it my balance is precarious, and that I have both scoliosis (a curvature of my spine) and dystonia (torsion in the region of my head and neck) made it very difficult and also dangerous for me to get on the scale and to stand in an upright position. The radiographer did not seem to know how to assist me. Fortunately, my physical therapist, who had accompanied me to the hospital and was permitted to be present in the examining room until the scan took place, was able to help me get on the scale.

In the report of the scan sent to my primary care physician, which she copied to me, I noted that my height was recorded as 59.1 inches. Although I know that osteoporosis can cause some loss of height, I doubt that I am now less than 5 feet tall—more than 4 inches shorter than I was when I was younger. Rather, it seems likely that this measurement was an artifact of my inability to stand erectly on the scale. I wonder why the radiographer did not think of using a retractable metal tape measure to take my height while I was lying flat on the x-ray table. But above all I am struck by the irony of the fact that the method used for ascertaining my weight and height could easily have resulted in my falling and fracturing some of the frail bones that the DEXA scan was intended to assess so my physician could make informed decisions about how to medically reduce that risk.

As I left the hospital, I stopped at the main information desk to ask whether there was someone with whom I could speak about a problem I had encountered during an examination procedure, and to whom I could make a constructive suggestion about how it might be rectified. The volunteer personnel behind the counter cordially referred me to a small room adjacent to the desk, where I was greeted by two other volunteers. I described to them the difficulties and hazards I had experienced in the course of my DEXA scan

---

[2] "DEXA (DXA) Scan—How It Is Performed." www.nhs.uk/Conditions/DEXA-scan/Pages/How-is-it-performed.aspx.

and proposed that the situation could be easily and inexpensively rectified by a decision on the part of the Radiology Department to purchase and use a different scale to weigh and measure the height of patients undergoing such scans. The sort of scale I had in mind, I said, would be like the one that my primary care physician (who had a staff appointment to this hospital) utilized in her private practice: a scale with a low, stationary step that was encased in a walker in a way that its handlebars could be gripped by patients to steady themselves as they mounted it.

The volunteers said they thought this was a good idea and took notes on what I said. It is unlikely that I will get to know firsthand whether they conveyed my suggestion to the Radiology Department or, if they did, whether my suggestion was acted on, because although the report recommended that I have a follow-up examination in 12 months, my physician did not think that the findings of the scan warranted another scan in the relatively near future.

* * *

The periodic visits that I make to my ophthalmologist, Dr. Gold, take place every six months, unless some acute problem involving my eyes calls for his more immediate attention. The set of procedures that I usually undergo in his office are standard ones, including my reading an eye chart to test my visual acuity, and his examining the structures of my eyes under high magnification with the use of a slit lamp (a binocular microscope). His attention is especially focused on the symptoms of the several chronic eye conditions associated with aging to which I am subject. These include dry eye syndrome, which occurs when the eye does not produce tears properly or when the tears are not of the correct consistency and evaporate too quickly; blepharitis, an inflammation of the eyelid margins which waxes and wanes over time; small drusen—tiny yellow or white accumulations of extracellular material—that have long been present in my eyes; and an occasional subconjunctival hemorrhage of my left eye that spontaneously resolves itself within a few weeks. These conditions cannot be cured, although they can be treated. In my case, fortunately, none of them has occurred in a form that is as yet a threat to my vision.

My appointments with Dr. Gold are among the least anxiety provoking of the visits that I make to doctors. Why this is so is not evident to me, especially considering how crucial my ocular health and vision are to all the reading that I do, to my vast correspondence and to the writing in which I am con-tinually engaged—particularly, at this time, writing these essays. That he greatly improved my vision, especially my perception of colors, a number of years ago by performing cataract surgery on both of my eyes (replacing the cloudy lenses in them with artificial intraocular ones) has contributed to the confidence that I feel in him. In addition, the quiet efficiency and competence with which he examines my eyes, his down-to-earth manner in recommending everyday treatments for them with eye drops and warm compresses, and the unspoken way in which he expresses his recognition both of the professional work that I do and the concomitants of aging with which I am dealing have a reassuring effect on me. In the course of my most recent appointment with him he conveyed such reassurance to me by his responsive and resourceful response to a small incident that occurred in connection with the usual slit lamp examination of my eyes. The exam requires the patient to place her forehead and chin against the rests on the front of the instrument. I was unable to do so on this visit because of the degree to which my difficulty in lifting my head and chin above a certain level had progressed. Dr. Gold quickly took note of this circumstance and without hesitation or comment calmly found an alternative way to examine the structures of my eyes.

* * *

By far, the most stressful medical visits I have recently experienced are those to an oral surgeon, Dr. Thiel, to whom I was referred by my dentist when I developed a painful ulcer on the right side of my lower gum. Dr. Thiel's initial examination revealed that the ulcer on my gum was not only large but had become infected in a way that had caused necrosis of the tissue and bone that surrounded it. To deal with the infection he prescribed an antibiotic (amoxicillin) to be taken every 12 hours for seven days; and he scheduled two successive appointments with me to carry out debridement procedures that involved cutting away the nonliving, necrotic tissue, bit by bit, to help the remaining living tissue adequately heal.

The ulcer, the infection, the debridement, the prolonged pain and discomfort in the affected area of my mouth, the difficulties in eating that ensued, and the many weeks of healing converged in a way that took a toll on my overall physical health and sense of well-being. I was not only surprised and perplexed by the magnitude and duration of my physical and psychological reactions to the treatment of the ulcer and its sequelae, but also chagrined that I had allowed such a relatively minor medical-dental occurrence to so disturb me.

This episode made me think of Hans Christian Andersen's literary fairy tale "The Princess and the Pea," a story about a prince having difficulty finding a wife who is a real princess. One stormy night a young woman who claims to be a princess seeks shelter in his castle. The prince's mother decides to test this claim by placing a pea in the bed offered to the guest for the night—a pea that is covered by 20 mattresses and 20 feather beds. In the morning, when her hosts ask her if she slept well, their guest tells them that she was kept awake all night by something hard in the bed that she is sure must have bruised her. The prince rejoices, because he assumes that only a genuine princess would be sensitive enough to feel a pea through all that bedding. The story ends with the couple's marriage and the assumption that the couple lived happily ever after.

I saw a resemblance between my response to a circumscribed mouth ulcer and its concomitants, on the one hand, and the hypersensitivity of the fabled princess to a pea, on the other. But I have no fairy-tale illusions about the source of my reactions. I know all too well that, realistically, my reactions are part of the "You-are-88-years-old" macro-diagnosis that my primary care physician once made.

Chapter 10

PLAGUES

Since March 2014, when an outbreak of Ebola first occurred in West Africa, I have intently followed the trajectory of this lethal and infectious hemorrhagic viral disease. At the time, Ebola could not be diagnosed until a person incubating it became clinically ill with symptoms including headaches, fever, malaise, a maculopapular rash, conjunctivitis and joint pains. There was not yet a preventive vaccine for Ebola, and the only way to stop its incidence was to break through the chains of transmission. Although progress has been made, there remains no therapeutic drug, and its origins are still not clearly understood.

Ebola spread exponentially in three West African countries—Guinea, Liberia and Sierra Leone—and became epidemic. The US Centers for Disease Control and Prevention (CDC), in conjunction with the World Health Organization (WHO), documented the number of people infected. By the end of October 2014, 13,676 persons in these three countries had contracted Ebola, and 4,910 of them had died. By mid-November, these figures were updated to 14,383 cases, with 5,165 deaths. "Limited transmission" of Ebola had also occurred in Nigeria (20 cases, with 1 death), in Spain (1 case, no deaths) and in the United States (4 cases, 1 death). Two "travel-associated" cases—one in Mali, and one in Senegal—occurred. In Mali, three other people developed Ebola, and all four people with the disease died. Concurrently with these outbreaks, but epidemiologically unrelated to them, a less virulent, more contained, strain of the virus emerged in the Equator region of the Democratic Republic of Congo. By late October, 38 laboratory-confirmed and 28 probable cases had been reported there, with a toll of 49 deaths. On October 17 and October 18 respectively, the outbreaks of Ebola in Nigeria and Senegal were declared over, when 42 days—constituting two 21-day incubation cycles of the virus—had elapsed in those locales since the last patient in isolation had become laboratory negative for the disease.

This was the 25th time that Ebola had occurred on the continent of Africa since its first known outbreak in Zaïre (now the Democratic Republic of Congo) in 1976. But the scope of the 2014 epidemic in West Africa, the rapidity with which it spread, and its mortality rate were unprecedented. It was the largest and deadliest Ebola outbreak on record. Only belatedly was there international recognition that this time the proportions to which Ebola had developed constituted a public health emergency and humanitarian crisis of global import—a delay that retrospectively was largely attributed to the shortsightedness and shortcomings of WHO.

The occurrence, spread and effects of Ebola, and the reactions to it, have evocative personal meaning for me. To begin with, they are associated with two of the milieus in which for many years I conducted firsthand sociological research: in Zaïre, and inside the international medical humanitarian organization Doctors Without Borders/Médecins Sans Frontières (MSF). Since the inception of the Ebola outbreak in Guinea in March 2014, MSF was on the ground in West Africa, providing most of the care for people who were stricken with the disease, while calling out to the world about the massive international mobilization of human and technical resources needed to cope with and curb an epidemic of this magnitude. About 3,400 MSF staff members were dealing with Ebola in West Africa, where by the end of October 2014 they were treating more than 60 percent of all Ebola patients. MSF sent more than 700 international ("expatriate") staff members to the region and operated 15 Ebola management centers and transit centers (as many as 8 of them simultaneously) in the three most affected countries. The centers provided approximately 600 beds in isolation units and admitted more than 5,600 patients, 3,500 of them diagnosed with Ebola, 1,400 of whom survived.

My own medical history also connects me with Ebola—most particularly through my experience as a patient with bulbar and spinal poliomyelitis in the mid-1940s, during a period when a polio epidemic occurred in some region of the United States virtually every summer. At that time, fear and panic dominated most communities. No medicine had succeeded in treating polio, no vaccine had been developed to prevent it or produce immunity to it, and its route of transmission was not understood.

Another way in which I feel linked to the Ebola scene is a rather ironic one. It conjures up for me vivid memories of the three decades after World War II when the imminent worldwide "conquest" of infectious diseases was hubristically heralded.

* * *

I followed the 2014 Ebola epidemic through the media's extensive coverage of it,[1] and in a small way I contributed to stories about its treatment and

---

[1] The *New York Times* reported that since late July, "more than 70 front-page Ebola stories have been published, carrying the bylines of nearly three dozen Times writers," and

significance. My book about Doctors Without Borders had just appeared,[2] and several journalists interviewed me about the attributes of MSF that I thought explained why they were the first responders to the Ebola crisis in West Africa and why they continued to be the primary medical aid group on the frontlines of battling the disease, its human ravages and its epidemic spread. The sources of information that helped me feel most in touch with what health-care workers, patients and their families in Ebola-stricken African countries were experiencing were not the media, however. Rather, the epidemic was illuminated for me in a personal way through MSF's blogs—and the detailed Ebola response update document that MSF circulated every week to its head-quarters, missions and partner sections—and also the emails that I received from members of MSF whom I personally know, and from Suzanne Mikanda, my close friend and long-ago research companion in the Democratic Republic of Congo.

Members of MSF described the "reality of the lives of people" in the three West African countries as "overwhelming." The epidemic was like "nothing I have ever had to deal with in my life," one wrote. They described "devastation, despair, and helplessness as whole families are wiped out," and the especially heartbreaking deaths of so many children. They noted that because the hospitals were filled with Ebola patients, more people were dying from other diseases that are normally treatable, like malaria, tuberculosis and HIV/AIDS. All this, they said, was taking place in societies pervaded by poverty, and whose pre-Ebola health-care systems were rudimentary and barely functional—in Liberia and Sierra Leone, partly as a consequence of years of civil war.

In their dispatches from the field, MSF staff depicted their workload as "extremely challenging, both physically and emotionally." They made reference to how intensely uncomfortable and depleting it was in high tropical temperatures to be encased in the personal protective gear that they were required to wear when they worked in the treatment centers—whole bodysuits with safety goggles, breathing masks, three pairs of gloves, plastic aprons and rubber boots. The heat and the gear combined to pose a risk of hyperthermia and dehydration and thus, regrettably, limited the intervals of time they could spend with Ebola patients. They expressed concern about whether in these circumstances they were giving patients optimal care. And they poignantly alluded to the fact that being swathed as they were restricted their ability to

---

that the paper had "produced more than 350 articles about Ebola this year." Margaret Sullivan, "Journalism in the Time of Ebola," *New York Times*, Sunday Review section (December 7, 2014): 8.

[2] Renée C. Fox, *Doctors Without Borders*.

touch patients and to comfort them by holding their hands when frightened patients entreated them to do so.[3] The staff's risk of contracting Ebola was mentioned in some of the MSF "voices from the field" dispatches, but it was not dramatized—even though 24 MSF workers had contracted Ebola, and 13 died from it.[4] Many of the "voices," however, noted that MSF had been "stretched to its limits" in dealing with the velocity and scope of the disease's deadly trajectory, and they expressed how anxious, stressed, angry and frustrated they felt, because of what they regarded as the inexcusable tardiness and inadequacy of the international community's response:

> How do we justify the global dragging of heels whilst thousands of persons die needlessly? […] The angry frustration bubbling under my skin. International powers continue to remain limp in their response. Big statements, big ideas, but little feet on the ground. This epidemic never needed explode, the fuse was in clear sight of everyone, slow motion and totally predictable.[5]

And yet, "amidst all the loss and suffering," an article posted on MSF South Africa's website affirmed, "there are stories of survival": "Today, out of all the patients cared for in MSF's projects in Guinea, Sierra Leone, and Liberia, we celebrate the one thousandth survivor."[6] A dispatch posted by an MSF physician working in Sierra Leone jubilantly reported that "a day of three miracles" had just occurred when "two of our sickest-ever patients were discharged, and a baby girl survived against all odds." She went on to describe the friendship group that had been formed by some of the women who had nearly recovered from Ebola and were waiting for a final negative test result

---

[3] Hilde de Clerck, in "Struggling to Contain the Ebola Epidemic in West Africa," MSF-USA. www.doctorswithoutborders.org/news-stories/voice-field/struggling-contain-ebola-epidemic-west-africa.

[4] "Twenty-one of those infected and all of those who have died were local, African employees," according to MSF data reported in David Gauthier Villars and Jeanne Whalen, "Ebola Crisis Stretches Doctors Without Borders' Means," *Wall Street Journal* (November 29–30, 2014): A6.

[5] "May the forceps be with you," Blog by Benjamin Black. Leaving to Return/Doctors Without Borders. blogs.msf.org/en/staff/blogs/may-the-forceps-be-with-you/leaving-to-return. In recognition of how stressful it was to be dealing with Ebola under existing conditions, MSF rotated the expatriate medical staff whom they sent into the field in West Africa every five to six weeks, rather than maintaining them there uninterruptedly for a longer period. MSF field assignments usually have a duration of at least six months.

[6] "My Son Is MSF's 1000th Survivor," October 21, 2014. Médecins Sans Frontières/Doctors Without Borders. www.doctorswithoutborders.org/article/liberia-my-son-msfs-1000th-ebola-survivor.

before being discharged: "They take baths together, tell jokes, run races along the corridor to keep fit, and dance together." "I danced along with them in my protective suit," she exclaimed.[7]

Furthermore, a physician who has been continually associated with MSF through most of his professional career and is currently working in South Africa informed me that MSF is "receiving an overwhelming number of candidates volunteering for Ebola fieldwork—many more than the number of postings we can provide." The volunteers were coming forward, in part because "everyone in the organization—even ones who had not worked for MSF in years—felt compelled to contribute and volunteer to go [where] 'comrades' are involved." "Solidarity between volunteers," as well as "solidarity with people in need" account for it, he said. Notwithstanding the kind of solidarity that makes MSF a "movement" and "not just an organization," he assured me that MSF continues in its "typical MSF self-critical style" to debate such issues as whether they waited too long before speaking up about the need for an Ebola vaccine to control an epidemic of this magnitude, and if so, why.

* * *

I received news about the occurrence of Ebola in the Democratic Republic of Congo from Suzanne Mikanda, who in her email communications always addresses me as "Yaya," the word for "older sister" in Lingala. Her first email about Ebola in the Congo was based on her observations in Kinshasa, where she lives. The news was conveyed to her by members of her family who resided in the Equator province where the Ebola cases were centered; she learned more information from bulletins issued by the Kinshasa office of the UN Secretariat's Bureau of Coordination of Humanitarian Affairs.[8]

She described the "panic" that ensued when the Congolese government first declared on August 24, 2014, that an outbreak of Ebola was occurring in the country—one that the UN bulletin stated was the seventh such outbreak to occur there since 1976 but that was "unrelated" to the epidemic taking place in West Africa.

---

[7] Monica Arend-Trujillo, "Ebola: 'Three Miracles' in Bo, Sierra Leone," MSF-USA, November 2014. https://www.doctorswithoutborders.org/what-we-do/news-stories/story/ebola-three-miracles-bo-sierra-leone.

[8] Suzanne writes to me in French. I have translated the information and explanations she shared with me into English. When I thanked her for the research about Ebola in the Congo that she had conducted on my behalf, she replied: "I always like to do research, and to share with, and receive from others, what I can. It always makes me happy, and helps me to move forward with what is presently happening in the world."

It was the Christian churches, more than the government, Suzanne related, that were protecting the members of their congregations—advising them to avoid greeting people by shaking hands with them, to frequently wash their hands with a medicinal soap called "Monganga," and to be careful not to buy food that had been exposed to flies. MSF responded immediately to the Ebola outbreak, she informed me, by sending in tons of relevant supplies and equipment, and opening two treatment centers in Lakolia and Boende in the Equator zone where Ebola had erupted. This swift response was facilitated because MSF has since 1981 been working in the Democratic of Republic of Congo where, at the end of 2012, it had as many as 2,782 staff members, and because its so-called *Pool d'Urgence Congo* (Congo Emergency Pool) plays an epidemiological monitoring, evaluation and intervention role in the country. But, she reported, it had been difficult to convince some members of the local population that because victims of Ebola are highly infectious when they die, and remain so for an indeterminate amount of time, it was imperative for their burial to be conducted quickly and in a way that did not transmit the virus to participants in the burial rituals. There are certain respects, Suzanne pointed out, in which traditional African cultural practices and the beliefs with which they are associated—most notably, the ritual washing of the deceased person's body by designated family members—run counter to the procedures for a safe burial. And so, "it has not always been easy to isolate and deal with the deceased. There have been instances in which families have come and seized the bodies, washed them, and buried them according to custom." This is not only because these practices are the traditional way of respecting and honoring the dead, Suzanne explained, but also because people believe that "evil spirits and witchcraft" underlie the occurrence of Ebola, and that there-fore, if the traditional procedures and rites are not observed, these spirits will be angered and will cause even more "misfortune and perturbation" to befall the community.

In mid-October 2014, Suzanne informed me that 66 cases of Ebola had been reported in the Democratic Republic of Congo, with 49 deaths. The physician in charge of dealing with Ebola in Boende had just announced over the national radio network, OKAPI, that no new cases of Ebola had occurred during the past 15 days, and that if no new cases occurred over a period of 42 days, the country could be declared free of Ebola.

The next email that I received from Suzanne brought the update that on November 15, the national minister of health had announced the probable end of Ebola in the Equator region. Nevertheless, he advised the popula-tion to continue to protect themselves by observing the prohibitions against touching when they greeted each other and against eating animals "hunted and killed in the forest" and the meat of monkeys and bats. Suzanne reported that some people were ignoring the admonition about what was dangerous to eat because, they said, this has been their food since the time of their ancestors. Still, Suzanne concluded, with regard to the overall Ebola situation, "light is beginning to appear [*La lumière bouge*]."

On November 21, WHO officially declared that Ebola had been eradicated from the Democratic Republic of Congo, where there had been no Ebola cases in 42 days.

Suzanne's concerns about the health situation in the Congo are not confined to Ebola. With a mixture of dismay and indignation, she has written to me in the past about the deplorable state of the capital city of Kinshasa. Its pervasive filthy and unsanitary conditions, she says, its infestation by mosquitoes, and its poorly functioning health-care system contribute to the high incidence of many forms of sickness among its population. In this connection, in her account to me about the Ebola situation, she mentioned that once again she had recently been felled by an attack of malaria, which she attributed to two factors: mosquitoes seem to "like me a lot" and the overall "dirtiness" of Kinshasa.

* * *

On October 23, 2014, a chain of events changed how medical professionals, public health experts, governmental and intergovernmental organizations, local and national US politicians, the media and the American public viewed the Ebola epidemic. Coincidentally, that evening I was scheduled to be one of four participants in a live panel discussion on "Principles, Ethics and Dilemmas: Becoming Doctors Without Borders." The discussion, co-organized by Doctors Without Borders and the Johns Hopkins University Press (publisher of my book about MSF), would take place in the auditorium of Public Television Station WHYY in Philadelphia. The chief panelist was expected to be Sophie Delaunay, who was then the executive director of MSF-USA. She did not make an appearance, however because, as the MSF Public and Internal Events Manager who had arranged the discussion quietly informed the other panelists, upon her arrival in Philadelphia she had immediately turned around and traveled back to her New York office when she received the news that an MSF physician, who had recently returned to that city from Guinea where he had been taking care of Ebola patients, had tested positive for the Ebola virus and had been rushed to Bellevue Hospital. In a non-officious way, the MSF events manager made it known to the panelists and to WHYY's behavioral health reporter, who was the moderator for our discussion, that the reason for Sophie Delaunay's absence would not be given to the assembled audience.

Notwithstanding MSF's discretion about communicating what had happened, by eight thirty that evening when, back in my apartment, I turned on CNN television news, the story of the MSF physician who had contracted Ebola was being dramatically telecast in a way that eclipsed all the other evening news. Since his arrival in New York on October 17, it was reported, this doctor—now identified as Craig Spencer, a 33-year-old emergency medicine physician associated with the New York–Presbyterian Hospital/ Columbia University Medical Center—had been jogging beside the Hudson River, riding the subway, taking a cab, bowling, frequenting a coffee stand and eating at a meatball shop. On the morning of October 23, the newscasts recounted, he developed a temperature of 101.3 and only then was transported to the special Ebola unit at Bellevue Hospital, where he was put in isolation.

The media stories that featured Dr. Spencer during the days that followed criticized him for failing to quarantine himself upon his return from Guinea rather than "running around" the city while he was "sick" and thereby potentially exposing many others to Ebola. In fact, however, Dr. Spencer was neither ill with Ebola nor contagious until he developed fever; even then, other people could only have been infected with the virus through contact with his body fluids. Furthermore, upon his reentry to the United States, he had gone through a debriefing process in MSF-USA's New York office, following which he had adhered to MSF's guidelines for staff members returning from Ebola-affected West Africa. Those guidelines included checking his temperature twice a day, finishing a regular course of malaria prophylaxis (because malaria symptoms can mimic those of Ebola), staying within four hours of a hospital that had isolation facilities, being continually aware of relevant Ebola symptoms, and immediately contacting the MSF-USA office if any such symptoms developed. In addition, he was abiding by the MSF recommendation to returning staff not to resume their professional work for 21 days—days in which to regain their energy and protect their health after the challenging and exhausting work they had done in the field.

The dramatically critical way in which the media presented the story about Dr. Spencer, and the misinformation about his contagious state that news stories contained, had the immediate effects of raising public anxiety about the imminent danger of a widespread outbreak of Ebola in the United States and of bringing politics and politicians onto the scene. The day after Dr. Spencer was hospitalized, New York governor Andrew Cuomo and New Jersey governor Chris Christie both announced the establishment of a mandatory 21-day quarantine in their respective states for all health-care workers returning from Ebola-affected countries in West Africa, irrespective of whether or not they had symptoms of Ebola on their arrival. The policies they instituted did not accord with those of the CDC or with the opinion of public health experts who, based on scientific and medical evidence, opposed mandatory quarantines. These experts were also concerned that enacting overly cautious, restrictive measures for anyone who had gone to West Africa to care for persons affected by Ebola, and the lack of recognition and esteem for them that these measures appeared to connote, might discourage other health professionals from volunteering. Volunteer professionals were greatly needed to control the Ebola epidemic at its African epicenter and to help keep Ebola from coming to our shores.

Governors Cuomo and Christie's mandatory 21-day quarantine policy for all persons entering the country through the John F. Kennedy and the Newark Liberty airports who had had contact with Ebola patients in Guinea, Liberia or Sierra Leone was immediately implemented when Kaci Hickox, a nurse who had been working with Doctors Without Borders to care for Ebola patients in Sierra Leone, landed at the Newark airport. There, immigration officials detained her for hours, took her temperature, which they erroneously considered it to be above normal, and transported her, under a police escort with sirens blaring, to University Hospital in Newark. When the physicians at the hospital took her temperature, it proved to be a normal 98.6. Furthermore, the results of the diagnostic medical tests that she underwent for the presence of the Ebola virus in her body demonstrated that she was not Ebola positive. Nevertheless, garbed in paper scrubs, she was initially put in an isolation tent on the hospital's grounds and subsequently was kept in quarantine within the hospital.

Kaci Hickox's experiences were even more histrionically reported by the media than Dr. Spencer's, partly because she chose to go public with them and "fight back"—portraying how she had been treated as "unacceptable," "inhumane," a "violation of [her] basic human rights," and a "big deterrent" to health-care workers' willingness to go to West Africa to treat Ebola patients. She also hired a lawyer who negotiated for her to be released from the hospital and permitted to travel home to Maine. Initially, Maine officials asked her voluntarily to quarantine herself in her house until November 10, by which 21 days would have passed since her last contact with Ebola patients; this arrangement, it was understood, would be involuntarily enforced if she resisted it. In the end, the chief judge for the Maine District Courts lifted this measure on the grounds that Ms. Hickox did not show symptoms of Ebola and therefore was not infectious. The judge's order required her to submit to daily monitoring for symptoms, however, and to coordinate her travel with state officials and notify them immediately if symptoms appeared—conditions to which she agreed. All the phases of her case were closely followed and prominently reported by journalists.

Ms. Hickox refrained from moving about in the small town where she lives, though she and her partner took a morning bike ride on a trail near her house—followed by a Maine state trooper and members of the press, including photographers. She did not develop Ebola.

Dr. Craig Spencer recovered from Ebola and was discharged from Bellevue Hospital on November 11, 2014. "While my case has garnered international attention," he said in his public statement at that time, "it is important to remember that my infection represents but a fraction of the more than 13,000 reported cases to date in West Africa—the center of the outbreak where families are being torn apart and communities destroyed":

> It is for this reason that I volunteered to work in Guinea with Doctors Without Borders. For over five weeks, I worked in an Ebola treatment center in Guéckédou, the epicenter of the outbreak.
>
> During this time, I cried as I held children who were not strong enough to survive the virus. But, I also experienced immense joy when patients we treated were cured and invited me into their family as a brother upon discharge. Within a week of my diagnosis, many of those same patients called my personal phone to wish me well and ask if there was any way they could contribute to my care. Most incredibly, I watched my Guinean colleagues, who have been on the front lines since day one and saw friends and family members die, continue to fight to save their communities with so much compassion and dignity. They are the heroes that we are not talking about.
>
> Please join me in turning our attention back to West Africa, and ensuring that medical volunteers and other aid workers do not face stigma and threats upon their return home. Volunteers need to be supported to help fight the outbreak at its source.[9]

Of his decision, after his recovery, to return to Guinea and its Ebola outbreak he said:

> I'm a doctor; I have experience working in really difficult situations—if not me, then who? That's why I went the first time. Before I left, I sat with my wife and said, "Look, there's a possibility I could get sick." We talked about it and made an action plan. When I got sick, we dealt with it. [Contracting Ebola] made me realize just how big of a problem it still

---

[9] "Statement from Dr. Craig Spencer," MSF-USA, November 2014. https://www.doctorswithoutborders.org/what-we-do/news-stories/news/statement-dr-craig-spencer.

is and that we needed more people to respond to it. So I sat down with my wife again and said, "I think I need to go back." I had worked in an Ebola treatment center for seven weeks and understood what happened within those walls. I knew my voice and my experience would allow me to be able to talk about the epidemic as a whole. MSF was really supportive, and so was my wife and family. They knew how much it meant to me.[10]

* * *

By the end of October 2014, a patchwork of rules and procedures for quarantining doctors, nurses and other health-care professionals returning to the United States from Ebola-stricken West African countries had developed on the American scene. The CDC held that mandatory quarantining for all medical workers coming back from Guinea, Liberia and Sierra Leone was not scientifically based or justified. But it advised that workers should monitor their health by taking their temperature daily, and that they should check in every day with a local health department official. In varying degrees, states such as Illinois and Florida, and also the District of Columbia, were following CDC guidelines. However, California, Connecticut, Georgia and Maine established stricter policies, along the lines of those in New Jersey and New York. And the Pentagon instituted the strictest policy of all: a mandatory 21-day quarantine on their home base for troops returning from the military's Ebola mission in West Africa.

In that month of October 2014, a Connecticut girl was barred from attending her elementary school because she had traveled to Nigeria with her parents to attend a family wedding.[11] This and similar incidents in the United States were evoked by the widespread anxiety over the imminent danger of contracting or transmitting Ebola. The executive director of the Liberian Ministers Association of Minnesota reported that congregants in that network of some fifty churches were being seen as carriers of a virus rather than as persons; several church members who were health-care workers had been

---

[10] Ashlea Halpern, "Coolest Travel Jobs: What It's Like to Work for Doctors Without Borders," *AFAR*, September 13, 2017. https://www.afar.com/magazine/coolest-travel-jobs-what-its-like-to-work-for-doctors-without-borders. More recently, while maintaining his position as director of Global Health in Emergency Medicine at the New York–Presbyterian/Columbia University Medical Center, Dr. Spencer undertook a three-month-long mission aboard MSF's boat *Aquarius*, rescuing and medically treating migrant refugees.

[11] Ariel Kaminer, "Girl 7, Barred from a Connecticut School over Ebola Concerns, Goes Back to Class," *New York Times* (November 1, 2014): A20.

"asked to go home from work after sneezing or coughing."[12] Researchers who had been in Guinea, Liberia or Sierra Leone in the three weeks before the American Society of Tropical Medicine and Hygiene's annual meeting took place in New Orleans were advised by the society not to come to the meeting because the Louisiana health department would quarantine them by confining them to their hotel rooms.[13] A Catholic bishop in Rochester, New York, forbade the priests in his diocese to travel to West Africa or other countries in Africa because of the "seriousness of the Ebola epidemic" and out of "pastoral concern for the people of God here in Rochester."[14] Some people working at Bellevue Hospital, where Dr. Craig Spencer was being cared for in its Ebola unit, were shunned or discriminated against outside the hospital. Even within the hospital, nurses caring for him in that unit noticed that staff members working on other services tried to keep as much physical distance as possible from them in elevators.[15]

* * *

My absorption in the unfolding of the Ebola epidemic reawakened some of my memories of the polio epidemics in the United States during my youth, and of my personal experiences as a polio patient. Among them are recollections of how fearful parents became about the danger of their children contracting the disease with the approach of each summer—the season of the year when epidemic outbreaks usually occurred. Although what caused the disease and how it was transmitted were not yet fully understood, parents anxiously tried to protect their children from polio by keeping them out of public swimming pools and movie theaters, ice cream parlors, soda fountains and restaurants that did not seem to be impeccably clean, and away from large public gatherings; by

---

[12] Minnesota has the largest Liberian immigrant population in the United States. Jennifer Maloney, Scott Calvert and Derek Kravitz, "For U.S. Liberians, Stigma Adds to Ebola's Burden," *Wall Street Journal*, October 20, 2014. www.wsj.com/articles/for-u-s-liberians-stigma-adds-to-ebolas-burden-1413830673.

[13] Jason Beaubien, "Ebola Researchers Banned from Medical Meeting in New Orleans," *npr shots*. www.npr.org/sections/health-shots/2014/10/30/360179428/ebola-researchers-banned-from-medical-meeting-in-new-orleans.

[14] David Andreatta, *Rochester (N.Y.) Democrat & Chronicle*, "New York Bishop Bans Priest Travel to West Africa," November 4, 2014. www.usatoday.com/story/news/nation/2014/11/04/bishop-ban-ebola-africa-travel/18461573/.

[15] Anemona Hartocollis and Nate Schweber, "Bellevue Employees Face Ebola at Work, and Stigma of It Everywhere," *International New York Times*, October 29, 2014. www.nytimes.com/2014/10/30/nyregion/bellevue-workers-worn-out-from-treating-ebola-patient-face-stigma-outside-hospital.html.

warning them not to use public toilets, public telephones or drinking fountains, or to buy food from street vendors; and by taking measures to keep them from becoming overly tired. Acting on the assumption that, especially during the hot summer months, urban areas were not as healthy as those that lay outside of cities, parents who could afford it sent their children to camps in the mountains or on lakes in the countryside, or arranged long family vacations at the seashore where the family could benefit from what were regarded as the fortifying properties of "fresh" ocean air.

The general public were not the only ones to react to the danger of polio with wariness and fear. Some members of the medical profession and some hospitals did, too. In connection with my own case, this attitude brought about a rather dramatic turn. On August 15, 1945, when our family physician responded to my parents' alarmed call to him about how progressively ill I was becoming by making a home visit to the apartment where I lived with my parents, he observed that, in addition to developing flaccid paralysis in my legs, I was having difficulty swallowing because the muscles in my throat did not seem to be functioning normally. His diagnosis was that I was succumbing to a life-threatening bulbospinal form of polio, which made it urgent to get me to a hospital as quickly as possible. That August 15 was V-J Day (Victory over Japan Day), which marked the end of World War II. The throngs of celebrating people made it difficult for an ambulance to wend its way through the streets and rapidly transport me to a hospital. But hospitalizing me involved a more fundamental problem: what our physician encountered was the reluctance of the New York City hospitals that he contacted to admit an acutely ill, highly infectious polio patient. In the end, through negotiations that I was too sick to follow, Sydenham Hospital in Harlem agreed to admit me.

Sydenham was founded in 1892 as a black hospital staffed by an all-white administration and white doctors and nurses. At the time that it agreed to admit me, although its patient population was still predominantly black, it had recently become the first US hospital to voluntarily adopt a fully desegregated interracial policy, naming African Americans to its board of trustees and to its medical and nursing staffs. My inpatient emergency care was immediately taken in hand by the hospital's white superintendent and his wife and a black nurse who, without donning protective masks or gloves, worked side by side to apply moist hot packs to my body that by this time was wracked by muscle spasms. The same black nurse kept vigil by my bedside all through the first night of my hospitalization. Putting her head beside mine on my pillow, she breathed every breath with me as my breathing and swallowing became more labored. It was because of her courageous willingness to expose herself to the contagiousness of polio in this way, and her extraordinary devotion to my care, that I survived that night.

When the National Foundation for Infantile Paralysis opened a special inpatient polio unit in Knickerbocker Hospital (located at 113th Street and Convent Avenue, not far from Sydenham), I was transferred there. I spent four months in that unit before I was discharged from the hospital to continue my convalescence in Florida with the home care of a physical therapist and a nurse. The term "quarantined" was never explicitly applied to the Knickerbocker polio unit, but in fact it consisted of an entire hospital floor whose occupants were all polio patients and the special team of health professionals recruited to care for and "rehabilitate" us. It was isolated from all the other services in the hospital. Some of our nurses occasionally related anecdotes about personnel from other floors trying to avoid contact with them. I don't know whether it was a formal policy, but the only visitors we had from the "outside-of-the-hospital world" were our parents. I have retained a poignant memory over the years of the one time that I saw my brother and sister during my long hospitalization, when they stood in the street directly below my hospital room and with the help of my physical therapist I was able to move close enough to its window to wave to them.

By the summer of 1946 I was reunited with my family. We vacationed together at Arrowhead Springs Hotel in San Bernardino, California, where my parents thought I might benefit from the dry, warm climate, the town's hot springs, and the hotel's outstanding swimming pool. It was a rather posh resort at the time, frequented by many Hollywood movie stars—a fact that delighted my young sister, who eagerly sought the autographs of the stars she recognized. I was still walking with the aid of crutches, and a number of the hotel guests seemed to know this was because I had had polio—knowledge that appeared to evoke as much anxiety as sympathy from some of them. The most notable encounter that my sister had in this connection occurred when she approached the table of a movie star who was breakfasting in the hotel's dining room and asked him for his autograph. He responded by drawing back in his chair, nervously inquiring whether I was "still contagious," and refusing to touch the autograph book and pen that my sister held out to him.

* * *

The other set of memories that the 2014 Ebola epidemic evoked are antithetical to my lived experiences as a polio patient. They are recollections of the euphoric optimism that prevailed among Western physicians and medical scientists in the 1950s, 1960s and 1970s about the progress that had been made toward eradicating from the face of the earth every infectious disease that affected human beings. The discovery, development and application of antibiotic drugs and of the Salk polio vaccine were viewed as milestones in reaching this victorious state. Peter Piot, the current director of the London School of Hygiene and Tropical Medicine, the first head of the Joint United Nations Program on AIDS (UNAIDS), and codiscoverer of the Ebola virus, has described how in 1974, when he was about to complete his medical school studies, he "broached the idea of specializing in infectious diseases" with his teachers. "The unanimous verdict of my professors," Piot has recounted, "was that I would be a fool to do so": "My professor of social medicine grabbed my shoulder firmly, to make sure I was paying attention. 'There's no future in infectious diseases,' he stated flatly, in a tone that bore no argument. 'They've all been solved.'"[16] The current era of so-called emerging, new and reemerging or resurging old infectious diseases in which Ebola has made its appearance was inconceivable at that time.

Cholera, malaria, HIV/AIDS, yellow fever, measles, tuberculosis, various strains of influenza, SARS (severe acute respiratory syndrome), MERS (Middle East respiratory syndrome), typhoid fever, West Nile virus, Lassa fever, Marburg virus (related to the Ebola virus) and, most recently, Zika virus are among the numerous currently occurring infectious epidemic diseases to which human beings are susceptible. Along with biological and biomedical factors—such as the genetic mutation of the viruses involved, and the development of drug-resistant forms of some of these diseases—climatic, economic, political, social and cultural factors contribute to their etiology and their spread. In addition, partly as a consequence of the overuse or misappropriate use of antibiotics, a significant increase in the incidence of serious, potentially fatal, infections with a bacterium called Clostridium difficile (or C. dif.) has been taking place in the United States. Furthermore, the risk of escalating occurrences of measles, malaria, tuberculosis and HIV/AIDS in Liberia, Guinea and Sierra Leone has been elevated because those countries have been focused on responding to the Ebola outbreak at the expense of other health-related activities.

I am mindful of the enormous progress that has been made in medical scientific knowledge and clinical medicine since 1945 when I was a 17-year-old polio patient, and I am aware that "the global initiative to eliminate poliomyelitis through vaccination has helped to reduce the number of cases by more than 99% in 30 years."[17] But polio is surging again in Pakistan where, during the first week of October 2014, "the country reported 202 cases of paralysis, the first time in 14 years the figure topped 200." These cases accounted for 85 percent

[16] Peter Piot (with Ruth Marshall), *No Time to Lose: A Life in Pursuit of Deadly Viruses* (New York: W. W. Norton, 2012), p. 6.

[17] "Vaccine-Resistant Polio Strain Discovered," *Science Daily*, November 4, 2014. www.sciencedaily.com/releases/2014/11/141104111408.htm.

of the world's polio cases. Polio vaccination has not taken place for several years in the North Waziristan region of Pakistan, where it has been banned by the Taliban, who have "killed some fifty vaccinators or their police escorts" since 2012; "as many as 350,000 unvaccinated children" who have been driven out of that area "now live in slums all over the country."[18] With its "ballooning polio case count," Pakistan also "constantly reinfects neighboring Afghanistan."[19] The incidence of polio is reported to have risen once more in Syria, too, partly as a breakdown in the medical and public health systems in that country. In addition, after two years with no cases of polio reported in Africa, two new cases of children with a paralytic form of polio were discovered in Borno State, Nigeria, in July 2016. That these children lived in different towns, that both of them had a strain of the virus that had been identified in Borno State five years earlier, and that only one of every two hundred cases of polio involves paralysis suggested that there might be many more "hidden cases."[20]

Furthermore, researchers have discovered a new vaccine-resistant polio strain with a DNA sequence that "shows two mutations, unknown until now, of the proteins that form the 'shell' (capsid) of the virus." The evolution of the virus "complicates the task for the antibodies produced by the immune system of the vaccinated patient as they can no longer recognize the viral strain."[21] The vaccine-resistant strain accounted for the "exceptionally high mortality rate" that occurred in an outbreak of polio in 2010 in the Republic of Congo. Of the 445 persons confirmed to have contracted polio, 210 persons died. Researchers' fears that other variants of the polio virus might emerge among populations immunized with the vaccine were realized in November 2014, when two cases of "vaccine-derived polio paralysis" caused by mutating polio vaccine were found in South Sudan, and one case in Madagascar.[22]

* * *

---

[18] Donald G. McNeil Jr., "Polio on the Rise Again in Pakistan, Officials Say," *International New York Times*, October 13, 2014. www.nytimes.com/2014/10/14/health/-polio-on-the-rise-again-in-pakistan-officials-say.html.

[19] Leslie Roberts, "Just One Poliovirus Left to Go?," *Science* 346, no. 6211 (November 14, 2014): 795.

[20] Donald G. McNeil Jr., "Polio Response in Africa to Be Fast, Difficult, and Possibly Dangerous," *New York Times*, August 12, 2016. www.nytimes.com/2016/08/13/health/polio-vaccination-africa-nigeria.html.

[21] "Vaccine-Resistant Polio Strain Discovered."

[22] Donald G. McNeil Jr., "Rare Vaccine-Derived Polio Discovered in Two Countries," *International New York Times*. www.nytimes.com/2014/11/15/world/africa/rare-vaccine-derived-polio-discovered-in-2-countries.html. The "vaccine-derived form is created when the attenuated virus used in the trivalent oral polio vaccine reverts to its virulent, transmissible form" (Roberts, "Just One Poliovirus Left to Go?").

By late 2014, the number of cases of Ebola was decreasing. However, the transmission of the disease continued steadily into 2015, and it was not until August that the incidence declined to numbers as low as three cases per week. As of mid-August 2015, nearly 28,000 cases had occurred,[23] with more than 11,000 deaths. Of the MSF staff members, 28 had become infected with the Ebola virus. Of these, 24 were national staff (they were indigenous to the country where they were working), among whom 14 persons died from the disease.[24] The possibility that transmission of Ebola could reignite still existed. But tentatively promising results with the clinical trial of a potentially effective Ebola vaccine—the Vesicular Stomatitis Virus–Ebola Virus Vaccine (VSV–ZEBOVC)—were reported. And MSF has taken the initiative of beginning to create a biobank and a data platform for the research and development of new anti-Ebola products and diagnostic tools.

As the 2014–2015 Ebola epidemic waned, what a *Lancet* medical journal article colorfully described as a "parade of global health specialists" assembled in a series of meetings to consider what accounted for the failure of WHO and the international community to appropriately and adequately respond to the outbreak of Ebola in West Africa, and how to better "prepare, detect, and respond to epidemic diseases in the future."[25]

On September 8, 2015, the Albert and Mary Lasker Foundation announced that its Lasker-Bloomberg Public Service Award would go to Médecins Sans Frontières/Doctors Without Borders for the "monumental" role they had played in fighting Ebola in West Africa, and for the frontline work in which they have been engaged over the course of many years in dealing with medical emergencies throughout the world. It is notable that the award citation included a statement that MSF's bold response and leadership in responding to the Ebola outbreak was a "duty" that "rightfully" should have been filled by the international community.[26]

* * *

[23] This figure includes probable and suspected cases as well as confirmed ones.

[24] Deane Marchbein, "The Response to Ebola—Looking Back and Looking Ahead: The 2015 Lasker-Bloomberg Public Service Award," *JAMA*, Published online September 8, 2015. http://jamanetwork.com/journals/jama/article-abstract/2436309.

[25] Richard Horton, "Offline: A Pervasive Failure to Learn the Lessons of Ebola," *The Lancet*. https://www.thelancet.com/journals/lancet/article/PIIS0140-6736(15)00152-X/fulltext.

[26] Denise Grady, "Lasker Prizes Given for Discoveries in Cancer and Genetics, and for Ebola Response," *New York Times*, September 8, 2015. www.nytimes.com/2015/09/09/health/lasker-awards-go-to-3-scientists-and-doctors-without-borders.html.

On January 14, 2016, WHO declared that the Ebola epidemic had ended. This was the date on which for the first time since the inception of the epidemic, Guinea, Liberia and Sierra Leone all reported zero cases of Ebola for at least 42 days. The announcement was accompanied by a mixture of affirmations about ending the epidemic and cautionary statements about not assuming that the work was done, but remaining "vigilant" to prevent new outbreaks.

One day later, on January 15, 2016, a death from Ebola in Sierra Leone was reported. A 22-year-old woman had died on January 12 in Magburaka, a village in the Tonkolili district of northern Sierra Leone. A test for Ebola, which was carried out two days after her death, was confirmed positive on January 14, only a few hours after WHO had announced that the spread of Ebola had been halted in West Africa.

* * *

Zika Virus "Spreading Explosively" in Americas, W.H.O. Says[27]
Zika Virus a Global Health Emergency, W.H.O. Says[28]
Concern over Zika Virus Grips the World[29]

While the Ebola epidemic was finally, though fitfully, ebbing away, these exclamatory headlines announced the emergence and epidemic spread of still another infectious disease—this one caused by the Zika virus that belongs to the Flaviviridae family of viruses associated with dengue, West Nile yellow fever and Japanese encephalitis, and that is transmitted by the *Aedes aegypti* genus of mosquito. The virus was first isolated in 1947 from a rhesus monkey in the Zika forest of Uganda,[30] and for decades it mainly affected monkeys in a narrowly restricted area of equatorial Africa and Asia. However, by 2007 it had appeared in the Federated States of Micronesia, where 185 suspected cases of

---

[27] Headline for an article by Sabrina Tavernise, *International New York Times*, January 28, 2016. www.nytimes.com/2016/01/29/health/zika-virus-spreading-explosively-in-americas-who-says.html.

[28] Headline for article by Sabrina Tavernise and Donald G. McNeil Jr., *International New York Times*, February 1, 2016. www.nytimes.com/2016/02/02/health/zika-virus-world-health-organization.html.

[29] "Concern over Zika Virus Grips the World" is the title of a special report by Udani Samarasekera and Marcia Triunfol in *The Lancet*, February 2, 2016. https://www.thelancet.com/journals/lancet/article/PIIS0140-6736(16)00257-9/fulltext?code=lancet-site.

[30] The first published communication about this "hitherto unrecorded virus" and how it was isolated is G. W. A. Dick, S. F. Kitchen and A. J. Haddow, "Zika Virus: Isolations and Serological Specificity," *Transactions of the Royal Society of Tropical Medicine and Hygiene* 46, no. 5 (September 1952): 509–20.

Zika affecting human beings were reported. Between 2013 and 2014, four other Pacific Island nations experienced large Zika outbreaks. In May 2015, the presence of Zika in the Americas was confirmed by WHO. By February 1, 2016, Zika virus transmission to human beings had been "reported in twenty-eight countries and territories, mainly in the Americas, including Brazil, Colombia, Venezuela, Mexico, Haiti and Barbados."[31] Dr. Anthony Fauci, Director of the US National Institute of Allergy and Infectious Diseases, characterized the Zika epidemic as "an unfolding story." "As with Ebola," he said, "this virus is something that could exist for years under the radar, and we don't know until we get thousands of cases what it really does. With Zika, we're seeing new twists and turns every week."[32]

On January 28, 2016, in a meeting with the Executive Board of WHO, Dr. Margaret Chan, who was then executive director of WHO, stated that the Zika virus was "spreading explosively" in the Americas, and that the level of alarm was "extremely high," especially because although most people infected with Zika develop a mild form of the disease that lasts only several days to a week, there was increasing concern that there might be a causal relationship between infection by the Zika virus and the disturbing number of infants in Brazil being born with microcephaly—a medical condition in which the circumference of the baby's head is smaller than normal at birth due to underdevelopment of the cerebral cortex of the brain and which can result in physical deformities and grave, lifelong cognitive and motor disabilities. (Another neurological disorder with which researchers began to suspect Zika might be linked was Guillain-Barré syndrome, which involves temporary whole-body paralysis in adults.) On February 1, 2016, WHO officially declared the Zika virus and its suspected link to birth defects to constitute an "international public health emergency." It is "an extraordinary event and public health threat to other parts of the world," Dr. Chan stated in a press conference, that requires an "international response […] to minimize the threat in infected countries and reduce risk of international spread."[33]

The next day, February 2, a case of Zika virus infection transmitted by semen through sexual relations, rather than by a mosquito bite, was discovered and reported in Texas, complicating the detection of Zika and prevention of

---

[31] Udani Samarasekera and Marcia Triunfol, "Concern over Zika Virus Grips the World," pp. 1–2.

[32] Quoted in Donald G. McNeil Jr., Simon Romero and Sabrina Tavernise, "How a Medical Mystery in Brazil Led Doctors to Zika," *New York Times*, February 7, 2016. www.nytimes.com/2016/02/07/health/zika-virus-brazil-how-it-spread-explained.html.

[33] Quoted in Sabrina Tavernise, "Zika Virus a Global Health Emergency, W.H.O. Says."

Zika outbreaks, and suggesting that safe-sex measures as well as mosquito control would be needed.[34]

* * *

"Less than a month ago, the world was celebrating the end of the Ebola outbreak. Now we are consumed by Zika," Victor Dzau, president of the US National Academy of Medicine, stated in a letter to the academy's membership on February 5, 2016. "The threat of infectious disease is ever-present, and its scale is enormous. We cannot continue to underestimate this threat," he stated vehemently. In his letter Dzau appealed to members to support the academy's "Global Health Risk Framework for the Future," which has been launched to "recommend reforms and measures to enable better preparedness and more effective governing and financing in response to global health crises in the future—especially to infectious disease crises and pandemic threats."

Six months later, on August 12, 2016, at the request of Alejandro Garcia Padilla, governor of Puerto Rico, US Secretary of Health and Human Services Sylvia Matthews Burwell declared a public health emergency in Puerto Rico due to the Zika virus, "which had infected at least 10,690 people […] among them 1,035 pregnant women."[35]

* * *

In September 2016, Mark Zuckerberg, the CEO and founder of Facebook, and his wife, pediatrician Dr. Priscilla Chan, announced their plans to invest three billion US dollars over the next ten years to "cure, prevent or manage all diseases by the end of the century […] within our children's lifetime." Their initiative will concentrate on the "four kinds of diseases that presently cause the most deaths in the world"—namely, infectious diseases as well as heart diseases, neurological diseases and cancer. They envision bringing engineers together with scientists to build new tools and technologies that they believe will accelerate breakthroughs in dealing definitively with these diseases.[36]

---

[34] Donald G. McNeil Jr. and Sabrina Tavernise, "Zika Infection Transmitted by Sex Reported in Texas," *International New York Times*, www.nytimes.com/2016/02/03/health/zika-sex-transmission-texas.html.

[35] Liz Szabo, "Health Emergency Declared in Puerto Rico due to Zika," *USA Today*, August 12, 2016. www.usatoday.com/story/news/2016/08/12/health-emergency-declared-puerto-rico-due-zika/88638014/.

[36] Brendan O'Malley, "Facebook Founder Ploughs $3bn into Disease Research," *University World News*, September 22, 2016, Global Edition. www.universityworldnews.com/article.php?story=20160922150440909.

Via email, I wrote about this project to Eric Goemaere, the physician who pioneered MSF's first HIV/AIDS program in South Africa and who is currently the HIV/TB Coordinator for MSF's Southern African Medical Unit. "Needless to say," he responded, "more investment in non-profit making R&D would help":

> But [...] it takes a combination of factors to eradicate a disease—from appropriate tools, [ranging] from vaccines, drugs, and diagnostics, to health services access, political willingness and human willingness. I'm not sure the Bill Gateses and Mark Zuckerbergs realize such complexity, preferring to focus on a technical "magic bullet" to do the trick. [...]
>
> Our humanity will inevitably be facing ongoing emerging and re-emerging infectious diseases [...] within an evermore interconnected world [...] making building preventive walls [...] completely unrealistic.

Goemaere's perspective is congruent with the persistence, the recurrence and the new outbreaks of infectious diseases that are continually taking place.

And indeed, in keeping with Goemaere's perspective, the measles virus was detected in 22 US states in the early months of 2019, and the number of measles cases in the country exceeded 700 by April 2019, the highest annual number recorded since the disease was declared eliminated in the United States in 2000. Among the milieus in which these outbreaks occurred were Orthodox Jewish communities in New York City and its suburbs, and in Michigan. Contributing to their occurrence were parental hesitancy about or delay in vaccinating their children, or refusing to do so for religious or philosophical reasons, or because of safety concerns.[37]

Although the annual death rate from AIDS and its new infection rates have fallen significantly, notwithstanding the millions of persons who are now on retroviral drugs, its incidence continues to be significant, particularly on the continent of Africa.

An effective vaccine has existed for yellow fever since 2016, but outbreaks of this viral hemorrhagic fever with a high fatality rate continue to take place in Africa and to a lesser extent in South America.

Polio no longer occurs in the United States, or in wealthy countries more generally. However, it persists in some impoverished regions of the world, and specifically in Afghanistan, Nigeria, Pakistan and Papua, New Guinea.

---

[37] Donald G. McNeil, Jr., "Measles Outbreak Infects 695, Highest Number since 2000," *New York Times*, https://www.nytimes.com/2019/04/24/health/measles-outbreaks-us.html.

Furthermore, in 2018, a polio-like illness, known as acute flaccid myelitis, struck children in 29 states in the United States.

In 2018, chiefly in Hyderabad, Pakistan, what was considered to be the world's first outbreak of a strain of virus that causes typhoid fever was experienced. It is resistant to the antibiotics ordinarily used to treat typhoid fever—and also resistant to other classes of drugs used to treat strains that are resistant to these antibiotics.

In addition, although a new Ebola vaccine has proven to be "highly effective" among the 110,000 persons in the Democratic Republic of Congo who have received it, the fact remains that the Ebola outbreak that began in that country in August 2018 is "second in size only to the massive Ebola epidemic that devastated three West African countries between 2014 and 2016."[38] On May 19, 2019, the *New York Times* devoted its front page to chronicling the situation in Beni, Democratic Republic of Congo, where politics, culture, war and history have combined in a devastating way with human misunderstanding. People with Ebola and grieving families and friends are suspicious about what is causing the disease to spread, and they trust neither the government nor the military. Men employed to bury the dead are threatened and attacked by mourners who accuse them of stealing body parts to sell. Those providing treatment, medical supplies, and vaccinations are also at risk: "When a doctor was killed, and treatment centers attacked by gunmen or set on fire, front-line health workers suspended their work, giving the virus time to spread. Some medical and aid groups have decided to pull some of their personnel from the very areas where Ebola has hit hardest." Mike Ryan, head of WHO's emergencies program, believes the epidemic can be stopped if—and it is a big if—a political solution to the region's violence can be agreed on.[39]

Like Goemaere, Anthony Fauci has characterized "the ongoing struggle between microbes and humans [as] a challenge that is perpetual."[40] "Winning," in his view, "does not mean stamping out every last disease, but rather getting out ahead of the next one."[41]

[38] Jon Cohen, "Ebola Outbreak Continues Despite Powerful Vaccine," *Science* 368, no. 6437 (April 19, 2019): 223.

[39] Joseph Goldstein, "Fighting Ebola When Mourners Fight the Responders," *New York Times*, May 19, 2019. https://www.nytimes.com/2019/05/19/world/africa/ebola-outbreak-congo.html?nl=todaysheadlines&emc=edit_th_190520.

[40] Anthony S. Fauci, "Emerging and Re-emerging Infectious Diseases: The Perpetual Challenge," 2005 Robert H. Ebert Memorial Lecture. www.milbank.org/publications/2005-robert-h-ebert-memorial-lecture-emerging-and-re-emerging-infectious-diseases-the-perpetual-challenge/.

[41] David M. Morens and Anthony S. Fauci, "Emerging Infectious Diseases: Threats to Human Health and Global Stability," *PLOS|Pathogens*, July 4, 2013. https://journals.plos.org/plospathogens/article?id=10.1371/journal.ppat.1003467.

My own perspective on infectious diseases is akin to Fauci's and Goemaere's. It is symbolically expressed in the conclusion to Albert Camus's allegorical novel, *The Plague*, which I have read many times over the course of the years.

When the inhabitants of Oran, the Algerian coastal town where the novel takes place, begin to celebrate their liberation from a deadly plague and the quarantine into which it forced them, Dr. Bernard Rieux, a physician who has witnessed and chronicled what the plague has entailed, decides to write a final account of it "to say simply what it is that one learns in the midst of such tribulations":

> However, he knew that this chronicle could not be a story of definitive victory. It could only be the record of what had to be done, and what, no doubt, would have to be done again, against this terror and its indefatigable weapon, despite their own personal hardships, by all men who, while not being saints, but refusing to give way to the pestilence, do their best to be doctors.
>
> Indeed, as he listened to the cries of joy that rose above the town, Rieux recalled that this joy was always under threat. He knew that this happy crowd was unaware of something that one can read in books, which is that the plague bacillus never dies or vanishes entirely, that it can remain dormant for dozens of years in furniture or clothing, that it waits patiently in bedrooms, cellars, trunks, handkerchiefs, and old papers, and that perhaps the day will come when, for the instruction or the misfortune of mankind, the plague will rouse its rats and send them to die in some well-contented city.[42]

---

[42] Albert Camus, *The Plague*, trans. Robin Buss, afterword by Tony Judt (London: Penguin Classics, 2013), pp. 237–38. *The Plague* was originally published in Paris, France, by Gallimard, in 1947, as *La Peste*. Goemaere, Fauci, and Camus each in his own way was prophetically realistic. As I am bringing this book to its hauntingly non-close close, measles recurrences in Europe and new outbreaks of Ebola in Africa are again on the front pages of the newspapers.

Chapter 11

MISS BALKEMA—AND MARYBETH

"Dear Dr. Fox: Thank you for taking a moment to read this letter," began the unexpected email. "My name is MaryBeth (Klinghagen) Thayer. Toinette Balkema was my great-aunt; my grandfather Clarence Balkema was her brother."

When my mother passed away in 2009 I received from her belongings the family archives. Since then, in between the events of everyday life, I have been putting together the pieces of family history.

I remember meeting Aunt Net, as we called her, shortly after my father was killed, in 1967. We lived with her in the Balkema family house […] for six months until Mom purchased a house of our own. I was 4 1/ 2 years old when this happened. […]

When I typed Aunt Net's name into the Google search engine, you can imagine my surprise [that] she was noted in two of your works. […] If it wouldn't be too much trouble, could you please "flesh out" just a bit your connection with Aunt Net and how she supported your work and research. Just a few details so there can be some additional information along with her name in the family history book.

The postal address at the end of the email indicated that MaryBeth Thayer lived in Kerkhoven, a community in Minnesota about which I knew nothing. The Wikipedia entry about Kerkhoven described it as a city with a land area of 0.82 square miles, located along US Route 12, approximately one hundred miles west of the Twin Cities region of Minneapolis/St. Paul, whose incorporation in 1881 was mainly due to the development of the railroad. The 2010 census set its population at 313 households, 210 families and 759 people, of whom 94.99 percent were white. The community was "home to" Lutheran, Baptist, Presbyterian and Evangelical Free churches. And the high school football team had won the state championship. The geographic and demographic ways in which the community of Kerkhoven differed from my urban and academic life in Philadelphia and my New York City origins were so great that both MaryBeth and I experienced our making contact with each other as an extraordinary event. "A part of me is still in awe of the connection we have made through Aunt Toinette/Miss Balkema via the Internet," she wrote to me after we talked on the telephone. "I shared the experience with my daughter," MaryBeth wrote. "Her response was, 'That is so cool. What were the chances of this ever happening?' My reply to her was that it was a miracle. And indeed, miracles come in all shapes and sizes."

* * *

Toinette Balkema—whom I always called "Miss Balkema"—was the person who played the most crucial role in my physical rehabilitation from the bulbospinal form of poliomyelitis that I contracted at the age of 17, which affected my spine and brain stem, paralyzed my entire body, and threatened my breathing and swallowing. She was the head physical therapist on the polio unit created by the National Foundation for Infantile Paralysis at the Knickerbocker Hospital in New York City where I was an inpatient for four months in 1945. When I was discharged from the hospital I was still in a frail state of health and capable only of taking a few steps with the help of forearm crutches. To protect me from the rigors of winter and advance my convalescence, my parents rented a small house for me in Miami, Florida, where I lived from December until June with Miss Balkema, who had accepted their request to care for me (along with a nurse) on a private basis.

At the inception of my relationship with Miss Balkema in the hospital I had been totally dependent on her for my ability to move. As my day-by-day, hands-on therapy with her proceeded within the framework of the Sister Kenny "muscle re-education" techniques on which her mode of treatment was based, I had worked intensively with her to identify, concentrate on and progressively activate and utilize the prime mover muscles of my body. From these interactions between us, and the interconnections between body, mind and spirit that they involved, more than a tactile, professional bond was created between therapist and patient. This bond was strengthened and deepened by the sequestered six-month-long, physical therapy–centered interlude that I spent with her in Florida.

* * *

When she entered and became a part of my life, Miss Balkema was in her early 50s. She was a sturdy and lithe woman, plainly dressed, with a smooth face, serene countenance, short, straight blonde hair and light-blue eyes, whose Dutch-American origins were physically discernible. She told me that she was a member of a large family of four brothers and two sisters and had grown up in Orange City, Iowa (the community of Orange City, named after William of Orange, was founded in 1870 as an agricultural colony by Dutch Americans from Pella, Iowa).[1] Churches—especially the Dutch Reformed Church—and schools were important entities in this small Midwestern prairie town, she said, and so was music. She described in detail the most important annual event in Orange City—its Tulip Festival in May, featuring a parade, Dutch costumes, wooden shoe–clad folk dancing and music including an evening concert by the Sioux City Symphony Orchestra. Miss Balkema alluded to her upbringing in the religious, Calvinist tradition of the Dutch Reformed Church, and to the wariness about Catholicism that had characterized the local church's outlook during her childhood. In this connection, with a mixture of amusement and rue, she described to me an experience she had shared with one of her brothers. At the end of a day when the two of them were hurrying to reach home before the sun set, she recounted, as they ran through an Iowa cornfield and darkness began to descend, they were both acutely afraid that "Catholics" might leap out at them from behind the tall, leafy stalks of the corn plants.

In a private, Christian, but unchurched way, Miss Balkema was a profoundly religious woman. She identified closely with Unity, a progressive, non-creedal, Christian, spiritual movement and organization, with respect for other faiths, that grew out of the late nineteenth-century American New Thought movement. Unity views religion as integrally related, practically as well as spiritually, to every aspect of life, including physical health and well-being, prosperity and happiness. Basic to its teachings are its beliefs in the power of affirmative thought and prayer, and in the inherent goodness of all people emanating from the spirit of God that lives in everyone. Much of the work of Unity is carried out through the numerous periodicals, pamphlets and books that it publishes.[2] Every month Miss Balkema received a pocket-sized magazine from Unity called *Daily Word,* which she shared with me in a nonproselytizing way, without engaging me in a discussion about its contents. Each issue was composed of an article, a poem,

---

[1] "Our Town," Larissa MacFarquhar's fascinating profile of Orange City, was published in *The New Yorker* (November 13, 2017): 57–65. https://www.newyorker.com/magazine/2017/11/13/where-the-small-town-american-dream-lives-on.

[2] For details about the history and attributes of Unity see "Unity School of Christianity," in Charles S. Braden, *Spirit in Rebellion: The Rise and Development of New Thought* (Dallas: Southern Methodist University Press, 1963 and 1987), pp. 233–63.

several short prayers and a devotional page for each day of the month that contained an affirmation, a comment or meditation upon it and a relevant verse from the Bible.

Unity's affirmative outlook on the power of positive thought and its emphasis on healing were highly compatible with the ethos of the Sister Kenny approach to polio treatment and rehabilitation that underlay the physical therapy in which Miss Balkema and I were interactively and collaboratively engaged. A project in which she involved me that grew out of these implicit shared premises was creating and updating a poster through which I expressed my aspirations for recovery and my goals for the resumption of a "normal" post-polio life. Because it was fashioned out of illustrations that Miss Balkema had me cut out of magazines and newspapers and paste onto its cardboard surface, the ongoing poster project also had the practical value of exercising and strengthening the muscles in my hands.

* * *

My knowledge of the details of Miss Balkema's professional career was sketchy. She had mentioned in passing that she had initially studied music. (Her grand-niece MaryBeth recently told me that Miss Balkema had a beautiful voice and, as an undergraduate at Oberlin College, she had been a music student). Rather than pursuing a career in music, however, she undertook training in nursing, and then in physical therapy. I knew that she was a graduate of the University of Iowa College of Nursing and that her physical therapy training had taken place in Boston in some unspecified department of Harvard Medical School. Because she spoke to me with admiration about Dr. Arthur Steindler, the founder of the clinical and academic orthopedic surgery programs at the University of Iowa in Iowa City and its head for more than thirty years, I was aware that she had worked under his direction as a physical therapist on his service. Her esteem for him seemed to be associated not only with his skill as a surgeon and commitment as a teacher, but also with the thousands of children who had a wide range of neuromuscular diseases and disorders, including polio, that he had treated nonoperatively as well as surgically; with his receptivity to some of Sister Kenny's techniques for treating polio—particularly the muscle pain and spasm it involved; with his broad interest and expertise in human body mechanics and movement; and with his role in helping to establish the statewide system to provide medical care for indigent patients.

Before becoming the head physical therapist on the Knickerbocker Hospital polio unit in New York City, Miss Balkema had been the chief physical therapist at the Children's Orthopedic Hospital in Seattle. During that period she traveled to the Sister Kenny Institute in Minneapolis to take a course that Sister Kenny was giving to nurses and physical therapists in her method of muscle reeducation for polio.[3]

I was reunited with my younger brother and sister when the 1945–46 school year was over, and together with our parents we traveled to the Arrowhead Springs Hotel, a spa resort in Sam Bernardino, California, where we spent the summer. Miss Balkema agreed to accompany us with the understanding that at the end of the summer she would join the physical therapy staff at the Rancho Los Amigos in Downey, California. At that time, Rancho Los Amigos was renowned for its team care and rehabilitation of polio patients, especially patients who were severely paralyzed and disabled by the disease and those who were in "iron lung" respirators. Among the shapers and leaders of this center was Dr. Jacquelin Perry, who, after serving as a physical therapist in the army, had become one of the first 10 women in the United States to be trained and certified as an orthopedic surgeon, was later recognized as the foremost expert on gait analysis and body mechanics in the country, and was one of those who first identified post-polio syndrome. (Rancho Los Amigos has become one of the largest, most comprehensive and highly rated medical rehabilitation centers in the United States. Now called Rancho Los Amigos National Rehabilitation Center, it functions under the auspices of the Los Angeles County Department of Health Services.)

Although I was eager to resume my college studies, the physicians caring for me felt that I did not yet have enough physical stamina or agility to return to Smith College where I would face the snow and ice of a Massachusetts winter. Arrangements were made for me to remain in the milder climate of southern California for the duration of the 1946–47 academic year, enrolled as a sophomore at Whittier College and boarding with a local family. Miss Balkema periodically drove from Downey to Whittier—a distance of 10 miles—to visit me, check on my well-being and give me physical therapy treatments. Those were the last times I saw her. We never met or spoke again.

* * *

---

[3] In *Polio Wars: Sister Kenny and the Golden Age of American Medicine* (New York: Oxford University Press, 2014), Naomi Rogers's historical work about Sister Kenny, her treatment for polio and her battles with the American medical profession about it, there is a reference to the letter that Toinette Balkema wrote to Sister Kenny on November 10, 1942, upon her return to Seattle after taking the course with her, in which Miss Balkema expressed the appreciative opinion that the Kenny "method of reeducation is completely reasonable, very satisfying and successful" (see p. 164 and fn. 103 on p. 179).

In retrospect, I am amazed, perplexed and also saddened by the realization that Miss Balkema and I did not maintain our relationship to each other over the ensuing years through correspondence. There is not a single letter from her in my copious files, and although I have always been a prolific correspondent, I do not remember writing letters to her. And yet, she is an enduringly important and beloved individual in my life, as the pages about her in my published auto-biography testify. She is the person to whom I attribute my physical and psychological healing and rehabilitation from polio, which made everything I was able to undertake after that paralyzing bout with illness possible.[4]

Through my email exchanges and telephone conversations with MaryBeth, it has become apparent that despite the lack of direct communication between us, Miss Balkema kept track of what I was doing. During her retirement years, when she returned to Orange City to live, she talked about me, and what she considered to be my professional accomplishments, to some of the members of her family frequently enough for them to think of me as "Renée." Phyllis, a cousin of MaryBeth's mother, remembers that Miss Balkema always had a photograph of me on her dresser. It seems that the "news" Miss Balkema had about me came chiefly from her correspondence with my parents, of which I was largely unaware. I do remember my father mentioning once that during the period when I was conducting sociological research in the Democratic Republic of Congo (then Zaïre) in the midst of turbulent conditions there, and he and my mother were worried about my safety, he had received a reassuring letter from Miss Balkema in which she affirmed that the work I was doing was important, and that she was certain I had the good sense and judgment not to take undue risks. She and some other members of her family must have had my parents' postal address because in my family files there is a letter that they received from her brother Clarence containing "A Memorial Record for the Relatives and Friends of Miss Toinette Balkema," with her date of birth (March 31, 1894), and her date of death (January 21, 1971). Accompanying this notice was a personal message to my parents:

Dear Mr. and Mrs. Fox:

Thank you for your continued remembrance of our sister and especially at Christmas time which is now past. She regretted very much not being able to send out cards but was made very happy in the receiving of them. We know that as you remember her from time to time you will remember her kind and loving personality and her desire to serve all.

---

[4] See especially pp. 44–50 in Renée C. Fox, *In the Field.*

She had great interest in Renée's work and future. Will you please let her know about her passing into her Eternal rest.

Sincerely,

C. E. Balkema

* * *

But what accounts for the fact that Miss Balkema and I did not write directly to each other? With a mixture of puzzlement and regret, I asked MaryBeth this question during one of our telephone conversations. Perhaps, MaryBeth said, she wanted to "let you continue to grow" and grow up in a way that was free of your relationship to her, and that would enable you to "be your own person." "Lovingly and willingly she returned you to your family and to your future. She did her part so that you could do your part."

A great deal of what Miss Balkema and I shared was never expressed in words, so it is conceivable that I subliminally understood and accepted why she neither wrote directly to me nor encouraged me to correspond with her. But it is only now, partly through the intermediary of MaryBeth, that I have begun to more fully grasp the import and the selflessness of the gift that she extended to me through her silence.

* * *

According to MaryBeth, Miss Balkema decided to spend her retirement years in Orange City partly in response to her younger sister Evelyn's invitation to come to live with her in the Balkema family house. After their mother died in 1950, Evelyn had moved into this house to care for their father until his death in 1956. MaryBeth described what she called "the Balkema house" with great appreciation. It was a wonderful three-story Victorian house, she said, built in 1907, with beautiful wooden colonnades and wooden floors, and a wide stair-case with a big stained glass window located halfway up the stairs that, because it faced to the west, was lit up every evening by the setting sun. During the time that Miss Balkema and Evelyn shared this house together as adults, two of their brothers—Clarence and Albert Junior, who lived virtually next door—visited every morning to have coffee with their sisters. The impression I have from MaryBeth is that until Evelyn died in 1967, although Miss Balkema no longer practiced physical therapy, and her daily round was more circumscribed by her family and the attributes of a small community than it had been in the past, she lived this phase of her retirement in lively good spirits and with a modicum of independence. Phyllis (MaryBeth's mother's cousin) told MaryBeth that her four daughters had loved "Aunt Net" because she was so optimistic and such fun to be with. And MaryBeth described her brother Jonathan as "entranced by Aunt Net" because she "embraced freedom," "did her own thing," was "a leading-edge person," and drove a Volkswagen Beetle. Not all the members of Miss Balkema's extended family viewed her this way, however, or understood the nature of her career as a physical therapist—its achievements and pioneering role with regard to the treatment of polio and the relationship between muscle memory and rehabilitation—or approvingly comprehended the nature of the life she had led in the world outside of Orange City. In her conversations with me, MaryBeth alluded to some relatives who thought that Miss Balkema was a nurse who had knowledge of massage therapy, and that she had espoused and utilized "Eastern medical techniques," which they considered to be scientifically and religiously dubious in character.

* * *

One month after Evelyn Balkema's death, MaryBeth's father was killed in the crash of a Piper Cub plane that occurred when one of the student pilots he was supervising failed to pull out of a required flat spin. The plane went down in an Alabama pine grove, killing her father and the two students he was instructing in his capacity as a civilian flight instructor. Under those circumstances, MaryBeth commented, her great-aunt Net probably thought that the right thing to do was to open the Balkema house of which she was now the sole occupant to her bereaved niece (MaryBeth's mother) and her children. MaryBeth and her sister Rachel and her brothers Jonathan and David (respectively 4, 14, 12 and 9 years old) and her mother moved into the house with Aunt Net until her mother purchased a house of her own six months later. The memories that MaryBeth has of Miss Balkema during that time are of a woman who was mourning the death of her sister and who, at the age of 71, was accustomed to a silent, structured, "almost reclusive" existence. MaryBeth described her Aunt Net's bedroom, located on the second floor of the house, as a "round turret, full of windows that faced the south, with a beautiful hardwood floor and furniture that spoke of the late 1800s. Tasteful but spartan." She remembers being surprised at being invited into her bedroom, "because I had been instructed that it was off limits." Aunt Net told her that in fact "her room was *not* off limits, but that it would be good to knock and ask before entering it."

* * *

Miss Balkema's obituary states that she had been ill for approximately five weeks preceding her death. That statement is associated with circumstances surrounding her death that deeply troubled some members of her family, among them MaryBeth's mother. The cause of Miss Balkema's death was breast cancer, for which she apparently did not seek medical treatment and about which she did not inform any members of her family until it had reached the advanced terminal stage that necessitated her admission to the hospital. MaryBeth still does not feel that she has a satisfactory explanation for how Miss Balkema chose to handle her illness. She speculatively wonders whether Aunt Net was trying to deal with the cancer using holistic medical methods that were premised on the connection between body, mind and spirit in health and in healing.

* * *

The family archives that MaryBeth inherited from her mother, the obligation that she felt to "flesh out" certain aspects of the family's history that the archives contained, the appearance of my name in association with Miss Balkema's in the Google-based search that she conducted in this connection, and the initial message that she sent to me brought MaryBeth and me into the kind of contact with each other that she likened to a "miracle." Although I consider the explanation for how and why our unlikely contact came to pass to be more mundane than MaryBeth has suggested, there are ways in which I have experienced it as an extraordinary happening. For, through the exchanges that have taken place between us, I have been transported to Orange City, Iowa, and Kerkhoven, Minnesota, been reunited with Miss Balkema, and learned more about Miss Balkema's origins, her family and how her life unfolded after we took leave of each other. I have also had the opportunity to enrich and to rectify in certain respects the knowledge and understanding her family had of her career and of her faith. And my own understanding of the meaning and magnitude of what I received from her has been enhanced. In the process, her grandniece Mary Beth and I have developed a strong relationship. "You, your friendship, your connection with my family cross my mind every day," MaryBeth wrote in one of her long emails to me: "I have carried a notebook with me wherever I have been, and have written to you a long, chatty letter about all the events and travel. And that is what friends do—carry each other in their hearts in whatever they are doing and wherever they are going. […] So be prepared—this isn't a short note—you'll be getting an earful."

* * *

Through our correspondence and telephone conversations, I have learned that MaryBeth is in her early 50s and has four children—three daughters and a son—and four grandchildren. Her mother, Evadeane Balkema, who was raised in a family that highly valued education, was a registered nurse. Her father, Simon H. Klinghagen, served in the US Air Force after high school graduation, after which he worked for the Northwestern Railroad and also attended Northwestern Bible College, whose president was Dr. Billy Graham. After marrying, Mary Beth's parents moved to Chicago so her father could attend Trinity Divinity School to become a pastor. Mary Beth told me that in 1957 they felt led to work with R. G. LeTourneau, a devout Christian business magnate, philanthropist and founder of the LeTourneau Christian University in Longview, Texas, who was a prolific inventor and manufacturer of earth-moving machinery. Her father worked as a missionary pilot in Peru in association with the company headed by LeTourneau. At that time, LeTourneau, Inc., was building a road through the Amazon jungle in Peru, developing the jungle land, and also engaging in "church planting" activities there. Subsequently, Mary Beth's father became the pastor of a Baptist church in a community in Alabama, which is where his death occurred in the fatal air crash with his student pilots.

Kerkhoven, the community in which MaryBeth and her husband now reside, is the town in which her father was raised. It is also where she met her husband when she was 18 years old—at a "mixer" at the Daily Vacation Bible School they were both attending during a period when she was seriously considering doing missionary work. She has great satisfaction living in her father's hometown, she told me, because she was a small child when he died, and inhabiting Kerkhoven has given her access to firsthand stories about him that have "filled in gaps" for her.

MaryBeth is an intelligent and insightful woman, endowed with an impressive array of gifts. She graduated college with training to be a medical assistant but has always wanted to be a writer. Her talent as a writer is apparent in the narrative accounts I have received from her about her Aunt Net, her own life and her family. For a while she worked on a local newspaper as a journalist, covering human interest stories, and won an award for the report that she wrote about "Ellie," a child who survived being born at just 25 weeks, weighing less than a pound—an event that MaryBeth attributed to the coming together of medical science and the deep faith in God of Ellie's parents. She is also an accomplished violinist and a pianist who, in March of every year, is the accompanist for students from the Kerkhoven-Murdock-Sunburg Public School who compete as vocalists in a solo and ensemble contest in which 10 high schools within a 100-mile radius of Benson, Minnesota, participate. However, as a young married woman who had four children within the space of seven years, she felt it was both an obligation and a necessity to undertake work that would supplement the income her husband earned as a truck driver. Neither writer nor musician was a practical career option under those circumstances. Instead, she drew on her handiwork abilities to earn money by crocheting, knitting and making patterns. Subsequently, her training as a medical assistant, supplemented by intensive library research, led her to become interested in herbs, natural oils and fragrances for healing and relaxation, which she developed into a small business. But her yearning to write persists, and several times in the course of our correspondence she has thanked me for what she alleges is "the encouragement" I have given her to "pick up the writing again and to pursue it fully." She has even referred to this as a "Godsend."

MaryBeth's deeply religious Christian faith pervades a number of the emails I have received from her—especially the one in which she described the crisis she underwent when, in connection with a broken leg, blood clots developed in her lungs and the physicians caring for her felt that her condition was so fragile that it would be too dangerous for them to try to fix her fracture or dissolve the clots. I had to "believe by faith" in God and Christ, she wrote to me, "that my broken leg would be whole, strong and straight without surgery or man's design," and "imagine and believe that the blood clots in my lungs were breaking down and that the blood would flow freely through my body via veins and arteries [...]. It was a season of faith and mind training for me." She saw a relationship between this and what I had described to her as the Sister Kenny–based method of muscle reeducation utilized by Miss Balkema, because it involved "working with patients and encouraging them to reach out in faith [...] calling certain muscle groups by name [...] and believing that [they] were working," MaryBeth wrote. "Oh, how I would love to talk to Aunt Net [about this] now!"

* * *

"I wish I could just go out the door, hop in the car, and drive a few miles to see you for the afternoon," Mary Beth wrote to me in April 2015, four months after our correspondence began:

We'd bundle up [...] and then go to a coffee shop and get our cups [...] along with a treat from the bakery. You would direct me to your favorite park. There in the park we would sip our coffee, nibble at our pastries, and bask in the sun's spring rays. The birds will be singing and we'll watch the squirrels dash to and fro. Perhaps a goose couple will pass by us and we'll toss them a few crumbs. We'll talk about little things, books we've read, people we've seen. We will be to each other a sounding board for the thoughts, ideas, and projects we have going. Best of all we will laugh together. And when the sun loses its heat, only then will we think about going home.

"There is a little park, less than a block away from my apartment house," I replied, "located in Rittenhouse Square":

> It was created by William Penn. It is graced with lovely old trees, blossoming bushes, squirrels, pigeons, a fountain, children at play, people of every age and many social backgrounds, strolling down its paths, conversing on its benches, sunning themselves on its lawns. There are no geese, though. But down the street there is a café called "La Colombe" that has the best coffee in the city, and delicious pastries that we could purchase before entering the park. So, if you ever make a visit to Philadelphia, this is where the afternoon we would spend together could take place.

"I marvel at how quickly our seemingly providential initial contact with each other has developed into an exceptional friendship," I mused—"a friendship that transcends historical time, geographical space, social backgrounds, and generations, and that has become very important to me. It emanates from the presence of Miss Balkema, your Aunt Net, in my life, and the blessing this constituted. What do you suppose she would think of the way in which you and I have become connected?"

In her next email to me MaryBeth replied: "I think Miss Balkema would think it was grand that we had found each other and I feel that she would want to have coffee with us if she could!"

Chapter 12

LIFE, DEATH AND UNCERTAINTY
IN PHYSICIANS' MEMOIRS

My abiding interest in matters related to the sociology of medicine led me to read five books in seriatim over the course of one winter:

- *Being Mortal: Medicine and What Matters in the End*, by Atul Gawande
- *When Breath Becomes Air*, by Paul Kalanithi
- *Do No Harm: Stories of Life, Death, and Brain Surgery*, by Henry Marsh
- *The Measure of Our Days: A Spiritual Exploration of Illness*, by Jerome Groopman
- *The Death of Cancer: After Fifty Years on the Front Lines of Medicine, a Pioneering Oncologist Reveals Why the War on Cancer Is Winnable—and How We Can Get There*, by Vincent T. DeVita Jr and Elizabeth DeVita-Raeburn[1]

The authors of these books are physicians.[2] Gawande is a general and endocrine surgeon, both Kalanithi and Marsh neurosurgeons. Groopman's medical practice and research have centered on cancer, blood diseases and HIV/AIDS. And DeVita is a physician and clinical researcher in the field of oncology. Kalanithi died in 2015 at the age of 37. Gawande is 51 years old. Groopman is 64. Marsh is 66, and DeVita 81. Each of their books is written narratively and movingly, as a memoir in the author's first-person voice, about what it is like inwardly as well as outwardly to be a physician who cares for the individuals who become his patients, diagnoses their medical problems, takes therapeutically intended action to deal with the problems, and makes prognostic

---

[1] *Being Mortal* (New York: Metropolitan Books, 2014); *When Breath Becomes Air* (New York: Random House, 2016); *Do No Harm* (New York: Thomas Dunne Books, Macmillan, 2015); *The Measure of Our Days* (New York: Penguin Books, 1998; published in 1997 as *The Measure of Our Days: New Beginnings at Life's End*, Viking Press); *The Death of Cancer* (New York: Sarah Crichton Books/Farrar, Straus and Giroux, 2015).

[2] Lucy Kalinithi, Paul Kalinithi's wife, who wrote the epilogue to his book, is also a physician—an internist. The coauthor of DeVita's book, Elizabeth DeVita-Raeburn, his daughter, is not a physician. She is a writer who has published in the fields of medicine, science and psychology.

predictions about the "natural history" evolution of his patients' conditions and the consequences of the measures he has undertaken to treat them.

What I found most striking about these five books, when viewed in relation to one another, is that, irrespective of the age differences of their physician-authors and their fields of medicine, or of what the reader glimpses of the differences in their personalities and social backgrounds, the major issues intrinsic to being a doctor with which they all grapple, and about which they vividly write, are identical. The shared spirit in which they do so is eloquently stated in the preface to Henry Marsh's book:

> This book is as much about failure as success, but it is not intended as a confession and instead is an attempt to give an honest account of what it is like to be a neurosurgeon. [...] I hope that the problems I describe will be familiar to doctors and patients everywhere. The book is also the story of an all-encompassing love affair, and an explanation of why it is such a privilege—although a very painful one—to be a neurosurgeon.[3]

Each of these physicians depicts practicing medicine as a demanding, challenging, absorbing and deeply fulfilling vocation that entails continuous, palpable contact with existential and moral issues of life and death and meaning. As Paul Kalanithi philosophically and poetically testifies, medicine enabled him to connect "the language of neurons, digestive tracts, and heartbeats," and of "brains and bodies," to "the language of life as experienced—of passion, of hunger, of love"—and to "the relationship between humans that undergird[s] meaning." It does so in a way that involves "directly experiencing life-and-death questions" and engaging in "moral action."[4]

The degree to which, and the ways in which, the authors are preoccupied with the deaths of patients for whom they have cared is striking in their accounts, as is their description of the process of dying.

On the last page of his book Vincent DeVita writes about the emails, letters and phone calls that he has received over the years from patients, among them those with Hodgkin's disease (a form of cancer that develops from the white cells in the body's lymphatic system) who were the subjects in the early trials he conducted with the first effective combination chemotherapy developed for that condition. Initially, he says, these communications "were about their survival and then, often, their marriages and the births of their children and years later, their grandchildren." He is profoundly thankful for these ongoing

---

[3] Marsh, *Do No Harm*, p. x.
[4] Kalanithi, *When Breath Becomes Air*, pp. 39, 43.

contacts. But he follows his expression of gratitude with a question that he admits he "rarely puts into words": "How can I tell these people, who reach out to me to share these lives, that while I remember them clearly and cherish their missives, it is the ones who are not here whose memory I carry with me most vividly?" It is with this haunted question that he ends his 381-page book.[5]

Jerome Groopman devotes an angst-ridden chapter to his patient "Matt," a boy with childhood leukemia who died from transfusion-conveyed AIDS superimposed on the underlying cancer of his body's blood-forming tissues. On the evening when Matt's death occurred, Groopman recounts, although he "knew that Matt was going to die, [and] that everything had been done for him that could be done," he was nonetheless stricken with "a deep sense of failure, of guilt":

> We, his doctors, had failed Matt, unable to save his young life, a life that five years ago had passed through the shadow of death and returned to a promising future. We had also failed the living. Billy had believed in us, his son's "expert Harvard physicians"; […] this faith in our abilities had not been fulfilled. Our science was not miraculous enough to change reality. I reminded myself that we were not gods, not able to perform the instant miracles needed to cure an incurable disease.

"Still," he continues, "I felt a profound sense of defeat, of loss," and this, in turn, raised Book of Job–like questions of meaning for him: "Why Matt Jenkins? Why after all he had gone through? […] I again looked for an explanation from God that cannot be seen in the world around us. I knew that I wouldn't find one."[6]

As its title and subtitle indicate, Atul Gawande's book is about our mortality and about physicians' and modern medicine's relationship to the inescapable facts that "we are all aging from the day we are born" and that our eventual, inevitable death is part of the "natural order of things"—of "the inexorability of our life cycle." We "live longer and better" now because of "scientific advances," he observes: "Increasingly large numbers of us get to live out a full life span and die of old age." However, he opines, this greater "scientific cap-ability" has "turned the processes of aging and dying into medical experiences […] managed by health care professionals. And we in the medical world have proved alarmingly unprepared for it."[7] "I learned a lot of things in medical

---

[5] DeVita Jr. and DeVita-Raeburn, *Death of Cancer*, p. 381.
[6] Groopman, *Measure of Our Days*, p. 110.
[7] Gawande, *Being Mortal*, pp. 8, 10, 6, 27, 6.

school," he concedes, "but mortality wasn't one of them"—even though the process of becoming a doctor began with dissecting a human cadaver:

> Although I was given a dry, leathery corpse to dissect in my first term, that was solely a way to learn about human anatomy. Our textbooks had almost nothing on aging or frailty or dying. The way we saw it, and the way our professors saw it, the purpose of medical schooling was to teach how to save lives, not how to tend to their demise. [...]
>
> Within a few years, when I came to experience surgical training and practice, I encountered patients forced to confront the realities of decline and mortality, and it did not take long to realize how unready I was to help them.

The core of Gawande's book consists of his firsthand exploration of what medicine and the medical profession in our society are doing, and are failing to do, to help us "deal with the trials of sickness, aging and mortality"—especially with regard to what he calls the kind of "sustenance of the soul" that would help us to make life "worth living [...] in our waning days," when we are "old and frail and unable to care for ourselves."[8] He recounts the conversations he had with elderly patients, the visits he made to nursing homes and to retirement and assisted living communities, and the discussions he had with a geriatrician, a critical care physician, an oncologist and a hospice nurse whom he also accompanied on their rounds. And in the final pages of his book he chronicles the trajectory of what he, his father (a surgeon, like Gawande) and his mother (also a physician) experienced when, in his early 70s, his father developed a spinal cord tumor that over the course of the next few years led to his death:

> We'd come to the same fork in the road I have seen scores of patients come to. [...] We were up against the unfixable. But we were desperate to believe that we weren't up against the unmanageable. Yet short of calling 911 the next time trouble hit, and letting the logic and momentum of medical solutions take over, what were we to do? Between the three of us we had 120 years of experience in medicine, but it seemed a mystery. It turned out to be an education.[9]

Paul Kalanithi's *When Breath Becomes Air* is a poignant and passionate autobiography of his imminent death and the process of dying that he underwent,

---

[8] Ibid., pp. 1, 3, 328, 77.
[9] Ibid., p. 223.

recounted in the dual capacities of physician wearing surgical scrubs and white coat and patient garbed in a blue hospital gown, with a plastic identification bracelet on his arm, who at the age of 36 was diagnosed with Stage IV lung cancer and who died of the disease when he was 37.[10] As his wife, Lucy Kalanithi, recounted in the epilogue to the book:

> During the last year of his life, Paul wrote relentlessly, fueled by purpose, motivated by a ticking clock. […]
>
> His book carries the urgency of racing against time, of having important things to say. Paul confronted death—examined it, wrestled with it, accepted it—as a physician and a patient. He wanted people to understand death and face their mortality. Dying in one's fourth decade is unusual now, but *dying* is not. […]
>
> He spent much of his life wrestling with the question of how to live a meaningful life, and his book explores that essential territory. […]
>
> Even while terminally ill, Paul was fully alive; despite physical collapse, he remained vigorous, open, full of hope not for an unlikely cure but for days that were full of purpose and meaning.[11]

* * *

All of these authors write with emotion about the kinds of medical uncertainty they face in caring for patients—and for Paul Kalanithi, in being simultaneously a physician and a patient. Prominent among them are the uncertainties associated with prognosis—with predicting what the outcome of the therapeutic measures that are taken to treat a patient's medical condition will be and, if the clinical situation is a grave one, predicting how much longer the patient will live. When the prognosis is grim, the basic rule these physicians try to follow in conveying information to patients and their families is to be honest, while leaving room for hope. One of the major problems they face in this regard is that the only kind of medical knowledge about chances of death and survival that exists is statistically probabilistic in nature. And so, as Paul Kalanithi writes, "The problem is that you can't tell an individual where she sits on the curve": "Will she die in six months or in sixty? I came to believe that it is irresponsible to be more precise than you can be accurate. Those apocryphal doctors who gave specific numbers ('The doctor told me

---

[10] Kalanithi, *When Breath Becomes Air*, pp. 1, 16.

[11] Lucy Kalanithi, "Epilogue," in Kalanithi, *When Breath Becomes Air*, pp. 214–15, 219.

I had six months to live'): Who were they, I wondered, and who taught them statistics?"[12]

In the chapter of *The Measure of Our Days* that Jerome Groopman devoted to the medical case history of "Elliott," one of his oldest and dearest friends, he describes the apprehension he felt when Elliott asked him, "What is your *choosh*, your sense, Jerry? Am I going to live?" (*Choosh*, Groopman explains to the reader, "is a Biblical Hebrew word [...] that speaks not of rational deliberation and assessment, but of inner vision").[13] Elliott had been diagnosed earlier with T-cell lymphoma and had been treated with an intensive chemotherapy regimen that resulted in the complete remission of the lymphoma but also, several years later, in leukemia as a consequence of the drugs, which had damaged the DNA of his normal bone marrow cells. Other than living with the leukemia, knowing that it would come back again even if it went into remission, Elliott's only choice was a bone marrow transplant from a compatible donor. If a matched donor was not found, receiving an unmatched transplant could result in a graft-versus-host disease reaction, which is usually fatal. Groopman responded to Elliott's question about what his *choosh* told him by saying, "My *choosh* is good. I believe you will make it, that you are going to live." Encouraged by Groopman's prediction, Elliott underwent a marrow transplant. It took place without complications and with remarkably positive results. But Groopman still remembers the trepidation he experienced immediately after answering Elliott's question with an "I believe you are going to live" prognosis. "I wondered if I had gone mad, whether [...] my rationality had collapsed and I was retreating into delusion": "Who was I to pretend to be a prophet, to have extrasensory perception? What did my *choosh* mean in clinical reality? Was I indulging myself and my closest friend in a convenient lie?"[14]

* * *

Groopman contends that "the deepest point of despair that a physician can reach [in] the nether world of uncertainty" concerns knowing whether or not a patient can be "reasonably sustained" and, if not, then "allowing" the death of that patient to take place, hopefully with a minimum of pain and suffering.[15]

---

[12] Kalanithi, *When Breath Becomes Air*, p. 95.
[13] Groopman, *Measure of Our Days*, p. 217.
[14] Ibid.
[15] Ibid., p. 160.

Henry Morse strongly agrees with this. In one of the most eloquent passages in *Do No Harm*, he declares:

> Just as it is irresistible to save a life, it is also very difficult to tell some-body that I cannot save them. […] The problem is made all the greater if I am not entirely certain. Few people outside medicine realize that what tortures doctors most is uncertainty, rather than the fact they often deal with people who are suffering or who are about to die. It is easy enough to let somebody die if one knows beyond doubt that they cannot be saved—if one is a decent doctor one will be sympathetic, but the situation is clear. This is life, and we all have to die sooner or later. It is when I do not know for certain whether I can help or not, or should help or not, that things become so difficult. […][16]

For Atul Gawande, this question arose when he "ventured beyond [his] surgical office" to follow some of his older patients "into their lives," and also explored the "transformation in elder care" that is taking place in our society. The insight that he gained from these extra-office explorations, he says, was that "as people's capacity wanes, whether through age or ill health, making their lives better often requires curbing our purely medical imperatives—resisting the urge to fiddle and fix and control." But, he added, "it posed a difficult question: When should we try to fix and when should we not?"[17]

* * *

The "Do No Harm" title that Morse chose for his book refers not only to a fundamental tenet of the Hippocratic Oath that physicians take when they embark on their medical careers.[18] It also alludes to another source of stress encountered by doctors about which each of the physician-authors writes—the potentially harmful iatrogenic side effects on patients of the procedures and medications that they wield. In this regard, Marsh recognizes the paradoxically

---

[16] Marsh, *Do No Harm*, p. 235.

[17] Gawande, *Being Mortal*, p. 149.

[18] It is believed that Hippocrates or one of his students wrote the Hippocratic Oath between the fifth and third centuries BC. It has been translated into many languages and modified numerous times. It seems that "First do no harm" does not appear in the original version of the oath, although the oath does contain the phrase "Also I will, according to my ability and judgment, prescribe a regimen for the health of the sick; but I will utterly reject harm and mischief." *Wikipedia*. https://en.wikipedia.org/wiki/Hippocratic_Oath.

dualistic nature of the brain surgery that he performs, which he describes as "controlled and altruistic violence" that involves deliberately wounding patients with the intent of therapeutically benefiting them.[19] DeVita's, Groopman's and Kalanithi's books contain vivid accounts of the side effects that many people with cancer experience from the toxic chemotherapeutic drugs they receive—effects that include great fatigue, nausea, vomiting, diarrhea, bleeding, fevers, infections, mouth blisters, skin sloughing and hair loss.

De Vita's perspective on the side effects differs notably from that of the other authors. He is a physician who has had a long and eminent career as an oncologist, who pioneered the use of combining chemotherapy drugs at high doses for the treatment of cancer, and who militantly believes we are "winning" what has been called the "war on cancer." He predicts that we are "heading for a time when we'll be able to cure almost all cancers. And those we can't cure as readily will be converted to chronic, manageable diseases." He describes himself as an aggressive doctor who will "do whatever it takes to cure patients, and if that isn't achievable keep them going as long as possible," and he views the iatrogenic concomitants of our present methods of treating cancer in this light. We must tolerate them for the time being because, he testifies, as in his own case, he has survived the "very aggressive prostate cancer" that he developed five years ago at the age of 75, through the use of "tools we already possessed […] and that will allow me to take advantage of new ones, should I need them": "To my good fortune, where we once had few, we now have many. There are more to come."[20]

* * *

While I was drafting this essay, I came across some strikingly relevant information in an article that I read about "the ethics of doctors writing about patients"—namely, that "the online bookseller Amazon offers 667 titles under the heading of 'medical memoir'"; that the "growing number of clinical experiences penned in medical journals as well as media outlets like the *New York Times* illustrates that physicians are writing about their experiences for publication and a wide and eager readership exists"; and that "blogs and social networking sites offer an expanding range of venues for publishing these narratives."[21]

---

[19] Marsh, *Do No Harm*, p. 76.
[20] DeVita Jr. and DeVita-Raeburn, *Death of Cancer*, pp. 255, 17, 297.
[21] Jay Baruch, "Physician/Writer: Dual and Dueling Responsibilities—The Ethics of Doctors Writing about Patients," *MEDPAGE TODAY: Public Health & Policy*, April 10, 2015. www.medpagetoday.com/PublicHealthPolicy/Ethics/50943.

Subsequently, I read a review of Paul Kalanithi's *When Breath Becomes Air* in the British medical journal *The Lancet*. In this review, Gabriel Weston, an English surgeon, commented that "A growing number of doctors—myself included—have picked up the pen in recent years, writing memoirs in response to what feels like an insatiable curiosity among the lay population to discover what it is that we medics are really made of." She characterized Kalanithi's book as "in a class of its own." "When I came to the end of the last flawless paragraph of *When Breath Becomes Air*," she wrote, "all I could do was turn to the first page and read the whole thing again. Searingly intelligent, beautifully written, and beyond that brave, I haven't been so marked by a book in years."[22]

Dr. Weston's reflections on this genre of book, and the deep impact that Kalanithi's memoir in particular had on her, made me wonder both why so many physicians are motivated to write such works, and why physicians and nonphysicians alike find such value in reading them. Is it partly because inside of the medical world physicians rarely talk with each other about the aspects of being a doctor that they feelingly narrate in their memoirs? And if so, what accounts for their mutual silence?

---

[22] Gabriel Weston, "Paul Kalanithi: Fathoming Humanity," *The Lancet* 367, no. 10023 (March 12, 2016): 1047. Dr. Weston's memoir, *Direct Red: A Surgeon's Story*, was published in London in 2009 by Jonathan Cape.

Part 4

ENCOUNTERS WITH CURRENT EVENTS

Chapter 13

TERRORIST BOMBINGS IN BRUSSELS

Unaccountably, I awoke a few minutes before 4:00 in the morning on Tuesday, March 22, 2016. I turned on my bedside radio, which is always tuned to WHYY, Philadelphia's public radio station. The voice that I heard was broadcasting from Brussels, Belgium, tensely reporting that at three seconds past 7:58 a.m., Belgian time, a terrorist bombing had occurred in the international departure hall of the Brussels airport in Zaventem, followed two seconds later by a second explosion there, and that at 9:11 a.m. a third explosion had taken place in the underground Maelbeek station of the Brussels metro rapid transit system, located close to the headquarters of the European Union. Including two suicide bombers, 34 persons died in the attacks at the airport, and 324 persons were injured. In the bombing of the metro station, 20 persons were killed and 106 injured.

These were coordinated terrorist attacks for which the Islamic State of Iraq and the Leven (ISIL) subsequently claimed responsibility. "It is hard to resist the symbolism of the Islamic State establishing a base for its murderous designs in the so-called capital of Europe at a time when the European idea is weaker than at any time since the 1950s," the journalist Roger Cohen opined in a piece published in the *New York Times* 13 days after the bombings. "Belgium as a state, and Belgium as the heart of the European Union, are as close to a vacuum as Europe offers these days."[1]

The perpetrators' identities were quickly established through airport and metro video surveillance cameras and eyewitness reports. The three airport bombers were Belgian nationals of Moroccan descent. Two of them blew themselves up after detonating the bombs. The third left the airport on foot and was apprehended several days later.

The driver of the taxi who had taken the three men to the airport recognized them from photographs conveyed by the media. He reported to the authorities that they had ordered a taxi by telephone the night before to take them to the

---

[1] Roger Cohen, "The Islamic State of Molenbeek," *New York Times*, April 11, 2016. www.nytimes.com/2016/04/12/opinion/the-islamic-state-of-molenbeek.html?mcubz=0.

airport in the morning. As instructed, he picked them up at an address located on a street in Schaerbeek, one of Brussels' municipalities. They emerged from an apartment loaded down with heavy baggage that they did not allow the driver to touch. After the airport bombings, police entered the apartment and found a stockpile of nails and screws, 15 kilograms of explosives, and 100 liters of acetone detonators.

Of the two terrorists who set off the bomb in the metro station, one was born in Sweden to Palestinian immigrant parents, and the other was a brother of one of the suicide bombers at Zaventem airport.

One of the terrorists seems to have played key roles as the likely bomb maker, making use of his electromechanical engineering training, and as the planner of the attacks. He and his brother had also been actively involved in the terrorist attacks in Paris on November 13–14, 2015, near the Stade de France in the suburb of Saint-Denis, and in a café, two restaurants, and a concert theatre in the city's 10th and 11th *arrondisements*.[2] Roger Cohen figured that at least 14 people tied to attacks in Paris and Brussels were "either Belgian or lived in Brussels."[3]

* * *

Zaventem airport and Schaerbeek ... How many times I had arrived at that airport and departed from it in my research-associated travels back and forth between the United States, Belgium, and the Democratic Republic of Congo (once the Belgian Congo) from 1959 to 1977! How vividly I also remember my visits at the beginning of the 1960s to the renowned Belgian drama- tist, poet, storyteller, and writer of epistles, Michel de Ghelderode, in the green-shuttered ground floor apartment on Rue Lefrancq in Schaerbeek, where he and his wife Jeanne lived.[4] And the unforgettable second letter that I received from him, written in his hand on parchment pages that came from

---

[2] Many of these details about the Brussels bombings and their perpetrators are drawn from the April 23–24, 2016, 32-page special collaborative issue of two Belgian newspapers— *Le Soir* and *De Standaard*—composed of interviews by journalists on their respective staffs with 70 witnesses to the attacks, their concomitants, and their immediate consequences. The persons interviewed included victims; medical first responders, police, firemen, and members of the military; airline, airport, and metro personnel; and members of local and national government institutions.

[3] Cohen, "Islamic State of Molenbeek."

[4] For an account of these visits, see "'Les Roses, Mademoiselle!' The Universe of Michel de Ghelderode," in Renée C. Fox, *In the Belgian Château: The Spirit and Culture of a European Society in an Age of Change* (Chicago: Ivan R. Dee, 1994), pp. 181–204.

Schaerbeek's archives, where de Ghelderode had previously been employed for some twenty years.[5]

At the time of de Ghelderode's death on April 1, 1962, Schaerbeek was still a district populated mainly by working-class Belgians. When I visited it again in 1987, however, many individuals and families of Moroccan, Turkish, and Algerian origin and Muslim persuasion were living there. As my taxi approached de Ghelderode's former house (now marked with a memorial plaque on its front wall in his honor), I passed numerous women on the streets wearing ankle-length dresses and Islamic head-scarves. Only two miles from Schaerbeek, the Molenbeek municipality of Brussels was developing into a community in which Moroccan Muslim inhabitants predominated. Demographic changes in these areas were a consequence of the large-scale immigration from Turkey and North Africa to Belgium that had begun during a period of economic pros-perity in the country in the mid-1960s, when the Belgian government had encouraged migrants from these regions to come to a country where factory and mining jobs awaited them. In 2016, some fifty years later, the Brussels bombings occurred in the midst of an economic slowdown. Molenbeek and Schaerbeek had become semi-ghettoized enclaves of second- and third-generation descendants of the original immigrants and were among the poorest areas in Belgium. In Molenbeek, "the second-poorest commune in the country, [...] 36 percent of people younger than 25 [were] unemployed."[6]

In this historical, socioeconomic, and sociocultural context, it is signifi-cant that although a "tiny minority of people who live in Molenbeek and Schaerbeek have any connection to or interest in terrorist organizations, [...] these neighborhoods, and others like them, have been targets for recruiting efforts by Islamist extremists": "An estimated 470 to 533 foreign fighters in Syria have roots in Belgium, the greatest number per capita of any country in the West. Many of those young jihadists have ties in Brussels and to Molenbeek or Schaerbeek."[7]

* * *

---

[5] Ibid., p. 184. I contributed this letter and the others that I received from him to the de Ghelderode collection in the Albert I Royal Library in Brussels.

[6] Cohen, "Islamic State of Molenbeek."

[7] Aaron Williams, Kaeti Hinck, Laris Karklis, Kevin Schaul and Stephanie Stamm, "How Two Brussels Neighborhoods Became 'a Breeding Ground' for Terror," *Washington Post*, April 1, 2016. www.washingtonpost.com/graphics/world/brussels-molenbeek-demographics/.

In several articles and in two of my books I have described in detail how I was drawn to Belgium on "inward and personal levels" and by some of the country's intriguing social and cultural attributes.[8] "I chose Belgium (or perhaps Belgium chose me)," I have written, partly "because its 'terrain' somehow coincide[d]"—psychologically, symbolically, and allegorically—"with my inner landscape." In those publications I chronicled the "transforming effects" that the many years of research I conducted in Belgium had on my life.[9]

The depth and duration of my relationship to Belgium, and the significance it has for me, amplified the shock and horror I felt when I heard that early morning news about the Brussels bombings. My first impulse was to make contact as quickly as I could with my closest friends and colleagues in Belgium. The rapid answers to the emails I sent were reassuring. Neither they nor members of their families or associates had been at the airport or in the metro when the bombings occurred. However, one of my Belgian friends wrote that his sister had had a "close call." He explained that she worked at the European Union "and walked out of the Maelbeek [metro] station exactly 11 minutes before the blast […]. She is still quite traumatized by what she witnessed."

The longest and most reflective response came from an emeritus professor of sociology, whose father and paternal grandfather had been senior civil servants. "For many persons it takes these kinds of horrible events for them to (re)discover the connections that they have with this small, so interesting, but sometimes unhappy country." "In general," he continued, "the commentary made by people and by the press is dignified":

> There has been no call for vengeance or for harsh repression […]. There is condemnation of these crimes and among certain people a desire to understand them that attributes their origin to the war in Syria, the terrorist strategy of Daesh, and the disorder in the world. Few people, other than some intellectuals, question the situation of our own society, the presence of an important immigrant community in Brussels, certain parts of which are captured by jihadist ideology. Those who think it is necessary to "understand" in looking for causes such as poverty, unemployment, [and] cultural exclusion forget that one is always

---

[8] See Renée C. Fox, "Journal Intime Belge/Intime Belgisch Dagboek," *Columbia University Forum* 5, no. 1 (Winter 1962): 11–18; "Medical Scientists in a Château," *Science* 136, no. 3515 (May 11, 1962): 476–83; "Why Belgium?," *European Journal of Sociology* 19, no. 2 (1978): 205–28; *In the Belgian Château;* and *In the Field.*

[9] Fox, *In the Field,* pp. 132 and 135–58.

responsible for these conditions and that all those who are excluded do not dispose of bombs in metros.....

It will take much time and political work to eradicate the jihadist ideology of European Islam, and that will entail considerable work by the Muslim community on itself. A sort of cultural revolution that must put it in phase with the reality of European societies in the twenty-first century [...]. The problem is also a European problem, because "Muslim" communities exist in France, in Germany, in the Netherlands, and in Belgium. It will be necessary then to attack this problem with much political intelligence and energy and many means. The difficulty will undoubtedly be to imagine new formulas.

[...]. I am happy that my parents were not witnesses to these horrors that totally contradict the ideas they had of our society. My generation (I was born in 1940) also has difficulty with this world, and above all I am worried about what the political scene will be for my grandchildren. We will have to leave simple representations of "globalization" to accept the idea that we are entering a very uncertain world threatened by many perils.

* * *

On April 4 I learned via the media that an eminent retired Belgian diplomat, André Adam, whom I had met under special circumstances in 1996 when he was serving as Belgium's ambassador to the United States,[10] had been among those killed at Brussels Zaventem airport on March 22.[11] His wife, Danielle, and daughter Isabelle were embarking on a trip to the United States that morning, and he had accompanied them to the airport. Their plane was scheduled to depart at 8:30 a.m. They were seated together, awaiting its boarding time, when the first bomb blast occurred, immediately followed by the second one, which exploded very close to them with such force that it threw them to the ground. "The ceiling fell on us," his wife recounted. "My hair was burned. My husband was curled up [...]. The last image I had of him," she said, was that of his being taken away by ambulance. She was severely wounded and underwent the amputation of one of

---

[10] André Adams served as ambassador to the United States from 1994 to 1998. He had a long and distinguished diplomatic career that included posts in Havana, Paris, Kinshasa, London, Brussels, Los Angeles, and Algiers, as well as Washington, DC. In the years 1998–2001, he served as the Belgian Permanent Representative to the United Nations, after which he retired from the diplomatic service.

[11] Jules Johnston, "Former Belgian Ambassador to US Killed in Brussels Attacks," *Politico*," March 16, 2016. www.politico.eu/article/brussels-attacks-us-dead-terror-facebook/.

her feet and was placed in an artificial coma for 15 days in the hospital where she was treated. Isabelle, the Adams's daughter, was unharmed.[12]

My one meeting with André Adam and his wife had taken place on March 8, 1996, in the Washington, DC, residence of the Belgian ambassador to the United States where, in a *vin d'honneur* [wine of honor] ceremony, Ambassador Adam presented me with the decoration of Chevalier (Knight) of the Order of Leopold II. "At the proposal of the Belgian Minister of Foreign Affairs," the honor had been granted to me by His Majesty Albert II, King of the Belgians. In the gracious remarks that the ambassador made on this occasion, he thanked me for the years of research I had devoted to Belgium, and especially for my book *In the Belgian Château*, which he characterized as a "remarkable, authentic and affectionate book about Belgium." He commended me for all the things about Belgium that I had discovered; for the wide gamut of Belgians whom I had come to know and had vividly portrayed; for my identification of the linguistic and religio-philosophical differences that were both integral to and rent Belgian society; and for my recognition of the attributes of Belgian life that transcended these differences and constituted what he referred to as the "Belgian-ness of Belgium." He also called attention to the sense of human comedy and the "qualities of heart" that pervaded the book, which he implied I shared with Belgians.[13]

It is with a mixture of continuing appreciation for what André Adam said when he conferred this honor on me; admiration for the fact that, during Adam's whole life (as Didier Reynders, Belgium's deputy prime minister and minister of foreign affairs, expressed it), his "professional engagement for the peaceful resolution of conflicts was striking":[14] and sorrowful indignation over the circumstances of his death that I remember him, his wife, and the occasion on which we met.

* * *

Along with responses from the Belgians with whom I am connected, many spontaneous messages arrived from friends, colleagues, and former students

---

[12] "André Adam, 79 ans, #EnMémoireBruxelles," *Le Monde*, April 28, 2016. www.lemonde. fr/europe/article/2016/04/28/andre-adam-72-ans-enmemoirebruxelles_4909924_ 3214.html.

[13] See "The 1990s: A Time of Consummation (I): 'Knighthood,'" in *In the Belgian Château*, pp. 339–42.

[14] "Honorary Ambassador André Adam Victim of 22 March Brussels Attacks." March 29, 2016. https://diplomatie.belgium.be/en/newsroom/news/2016/honorary_ambassador_andre_adam_victim_22_march_brussels_attacks.

in the United States about the Brussels bombings immediately after they occurred. All of them expressed great distress and sadness over the terrorist attacks, and worry about the safety and well-being of my friends and their families in Belgium. "You must be even more upset than the rest of us," one wrote, because of how "deeply immersed you have been in Belgium." "So much of you is related to Belgium," one remarked while making reference to my book *In the Belgian Château* and to my autobiography, *In the Field*, whose chapters about Belgium he said he was rereading. I was touched by their concern about how I was reacting to the bombings, and gratified that what I had conveyed to them about Belgium through my teaching and writing and in personal conversations seemed to have contributed to their sustained interest in that country and their humane sense of identification with its people.

* * *

On May 2, 2016, a close Belgian friend who is a member of Médecins Sans Frontières (MSF) and is currently posted in South Africa sent me his impressions of the state in which he found Brussels on a trip to Belgium from which he had just returned. He described it as "a city slowly recovering from trauma":

> Needless to say, the Brussels airport departure hall has been severely damaged. […] You do not see much upon arrival, but departure is completely perturbed, using temporary tents to register passengers, creating endless queues. Security control at each step, with more X-ray screening, and more body searches than ever […].

> Probably the most damage I could see at the airport but also in the metro and [on] all main streets [is] the ongoing presence of machine gun–armed military personnel, which I personally find very disturbing, knowing how useless it can be as a deterrent, while it seems reassuring so [is] welcomed by the majority. [I] am really afraid this might become "normal," [especially if] a right-wing government prone to extend the emergency state [came to power …].[15]

> Used the metro a couple of times and passed by Maelbeek station, which is also badly damaged. The metro was full and I actually found people more talkative, as if this created a new sense of solidarity.

---

[15] At the time I received this message, politically far-right developments that seemed to be gaining momentum were taking place in numerous European countries, including Austria, France, Denmark, Finland, Norway and the Netherlands.

In a nutshell I would say that most Brussels inhabitants are keen to demonstrate that life goes on for them as normal.

Tourists are dramatically missing. Restaurants and cafés mostly around [the center of the city] are completely deserted.

More concerning, I heard from some of my MSF colleagues, not [inclined to be] xenophobes, that it was better not to walk alone anymore in some areas of Brussels, even in full daylight. I did not have time to check this myself, but it suggests some areas have become some sort of ghettos, expressions of social disintegration never heard of before in Belgium […].

I used to consider Brussels (where I was born, so this is completely subjective) as the world capital of integration. [I'm] afraid this is probably not the case anymore.

Chapter 14

THE 2016 PRESIDENTIAL ELECTION

On November 8, 2016, I received an exuberant email message with the subject line "Election Day!"—punctuated with an exclamation mark—from my grandnephew, Leopold, who was then a senior at the University of Pennsylvania:

Hi, Renée,

I hope that you are excited on this historic day. I was at the [Democratic rally] event in downtown Philadelphia [at Liberty Hall last night] and it was just spectacular. It was an amazing experience to see Bill Clinton, and to hear Michelle, Barack, and Hillary speak. There must have been 50,000 people there. I voted at 8am, and then I got to meet Joe Biden who was on campus. [...] I attach a photo that I took with him. I thanked him for his work these last 8 years and his efforts to fight cancer.[1]

Let's hope we win!

Love, Leopold

The photograph that Leopold sent me depicted him and Joe Biden with broad smiles on their faces, standing shoulder-to-shoulder on Locust Walk of Penn's campus, firmly clasping right hands.

"How are you faring?," I wrote to Leopold once it became clear that Trump had won the election. "It was like a dream shattered," he replied, and he described virtually "everyone on campus crying" when they first learned of the outcome. With touching empathy for me personally, he expressed regret (implicitly because of my age) that I would not get to see a woman

---

[1] One of Vice President Joseph Biden's granddaughters was a freshman at the University of Pennsylvania, which probably contributed to his being available to appear on Penn's campus on Election Day. Leopold's expression of gratitude to Biden for his "efforts to fight cancer" was personally connected with the fact that his father—my nephew—had a bout with a leukemic form of cancer. All signs indicate, fortunately, that he has been cured.

elected president of the United States. But "I'm doing alright now," he said, "as I think I have gotten over the shock of the election": "Now I am waiting carefully as he assembles his administration. [...] It's very scary some of the names being considered for key positions in our government. I hope that the Democrats can resist his worst ideas and we will survive these four years."

"These *are* difficult, worrisome, and even frightening times," I responded, "but I have hope and confidence in your generation, the action in which you will engage, and the way that you will lives your lives." I mentioned that I was looking forward to framing the photo of Leopold and Vice President Joe Biden and placing it near the desk in my study, and that looking at it while I work "will greatly raise my spirits."

* * *

Over the course of the next weeks I received an outpouring of telephone and email messages about the results of the election from friends, colleagues and former students, and from a number of young professionals whom I am currently mentoring. Most of them expressed shocked dismay at the results and great worry about the state of the country. From teachers, parents and grandparents, I heard deep concern about how their students and their progeny would react, and about the future of these young people:

> Such a pleasure having a conversation with you, as always. [But] what a night followed. [...] It was incredible watching three quarters of the US map fill in with red, even though Hilary won more of the popular vote. [...] This morning, [our son] told [our granddaughter] that Donald Trump was our new President. She said (age 3 1/2), "Donald Trump is not a nice man."

> I am in a state of shock regarding the election results and it will take quite a while before I start feeling a bit normal. I will be in touch. [...]

> I fear for [my son] and for my students. The country in which they will live will be much diminished.

> Still in shock so it's hard to find words. I have not yet been able to read news coverage. And not yet sleeping well. [...] Important to remember that many students voted for the first time ever on Tuesday so that makes the outcome more difficult.

> We are on our way to spend the day with the kids. Hard to know how to comfort them.

Several of the persons who telephoned me right after the election were particularly concerned about Trump's plans to tighten immigration laws and deport immigrant residents—and they were especially concerned about the threat to the security and well-being of the "undocumented" children of immigrant parents currently enrolled in colleges and universities whom they are teaching, or who are among the pediatric patients for whom they are medically caring.

* * *

As soon as they learned the outcome of the election, friends and colleagues from countries outside the United States—including Canada, England, Belgium, France, the Democratic Republic of Congo, South Africa, India and Pakistan—also filled my email inbox with distraught messages. Virtually all of them expressed incredulity and perplexity, as well as distress and sadness, that in a country they viewed as the embodiment of democratic institutions and humane, universalistic values, someone with Donald Trump's attributes had been elected president of the United States. They were worried about international as well as national consequences. On a more personal level, they were also concerned about its impact on me, they said. They extended a mixture of support and condolences and voiced the need to continue to examine with me the explanation for what they considered to be a traumatic event. And they urged me to take what action I could to help ensure that the United States lived up to its vital humanitarian commitments:

> I woke this morning and felt sick at the news—as sick or more than I did on the morning of Brexit. What a world we have come to live in. I am so sorry for you. All that one can hope is that the Republican grandees take Trump in hand and advise and educate him, so that Trump in the White House is different from Trump on the loose.

> This short mail just to say you were one of the first persons I was thinking of when reading US election results yesterday morning. […] Just wanted you to know that I am thinking of you in these difficult moments. […]

> I know that in East and West coast [US] cities there was demonstrating all over the place yesterday night. But still I would like to encourage you to […] write a passionate opinion piece […] on the duty to keep U.S. commitments—in priority the ones on controlling diseases, [especially] HIV and TB. Doctors Without Borders does not take U.S. money, as you know, but we are very well placed to know what human disaster this pulling out could create.

> Tuesday, late night when the results began to roll in was early Wednesday morning in [Pakistan]. And so [in our center] we were (periodically) glued to the TV in Aamir's office. Watching as the electoral votes from State after State after State begin to pile up for Trump. […] It was both a

surreal and distressing experience, especially for me, to imagine this man at the helm of American affairs. […] I mourn with you.

I don't know what to say. I've never been so disturbed and upset about US elections. I had a nightmare on election night that I walked around in what seemed to be some kind of church, and noticed all these people piously but somewhat triumphantly (or perhaps Trumphantly) smiling, and I felt like shaking them up and yelling to them, "Do you realize what you just did?"

You have seen many more elections. Perhaps you have a wiser, more comforting view from an historical perspective. But I can imagine that you are as a US citizen even more directly troubled that a vile, cynical man who utters racist, misogynous, hate-filled insults as if it is just a normal way of doing politics, gets elected as the president of the most powerful western democracy. […]

Let us hope that as a minimum, the democratic institutions in the US are strong enough to control the completely unpredictable temperament of this troubling man.

The only positive comments on the election that I received from abroad came from my closest friend in the Democratic Republic of Congo, Suzanne Mikanda.[2] "Congratulations on the election of your new president," she declared in the first email that she sent me. "We have watched attentively on November 8 in order to live this great event with you. May the Holy Spirit help him achieve all that [Trump] has promised. And may God also help us to have the same good fortune. […] We greatly appreciate the respect for organization" that characterized the election, with "all becoming automatic," and "its dignity," she continued. "We dream of becoming like that."[3]

---

[2] For more details about Suzanne Mikanda and our relationship, see the "Plagues" essay. The quoted passages from her emails to me were written in French by Suzanne and translated by me.

[3] What Suzanne was implicitly referring to was that, in contrast to the American political situation, the president of the Democratic Republic of Congo, Joseph Kabila, whose two terms in office constitutionally ended on December 19, 2016, did not step down. Rather, he announced that elections would be delayed until April 2018, and that he would stay in power as head of an interim government at least until then. Protest demonstrations erupted in Kinshasa, the Congo's capitol, and in other cities of the country, to which Kabila responded by blocking radio, television and social media sites, and by unleashing his security forces on the demonstrations, with the result that, according to a Human Rights Watch report, "at least 34 people were killed and at least 275 people were arrested in one day." The repercussions of these events threatened to ignite further widespread violence in a country that has been continually faced with internal wars and rebel

Notwithstanding Suzanne's appreciation of the comparatively orderly, legal and efficient conduct of the election in the United States, a follow-up email that I received from her made it clear that she was not completely satisfied with its outcome. "I am continuing to think of you," she wrote, "above all in attentively following the criticisms of the elections in the USA. Truly, [...] we liked Madame [Clinton] more, and the young people [among us] say that [she lost] because men do not like having women at the head. [...] In Europe they don't appreciate Donald either."

The message that I received from a senior Belgian social scientist came closest to my own perspective on the larger-than-American implications of Trump's election. "Like you," he wrote, "I feel that the period we are going through is very somber and that there are not many public grounds for rejoicing":

The Middle East, ravaged by violence for decades, continues to be an abscess of painful fixation for the entire world. [...] Corresponding in Europe to the election of Mr. Trump in the United States are Brexit, the rise of narrow forms of nationalism in various countries, [and] the degradation of the democratic ideal. [...] I fear that we may be at the beginning of a process that is undoing the Post World War II world order. [...]

The election of Mr. Trump remains perplexing, even though there are good analysts to explain this vote as a rejection of the political establishment. The same phenomenon exists in France with the National Front vote. [...] History has shown us, alas, how populism that feeds on all the failures of democracy, never provides solutions to the problems that it denounces, but to the contrary, is the bearer of political violence, exclusion and repression. What is happening in Hungary and also in Poland is an unhappy example in this regard with the promulgation of laws that restrict freedom, the reduction of freedom of the press, and other very problematic matters. [...]

With regard to your country, I strongly hope that Mr. Trump will be "controlled" by Congress, the press, and his own party. The problem is that there is a strong risk that this control [will be] exerted to deal with internal matters and not with external polity matters in which [Trump] is totally and dangerously illiterate.[4]

* * *

---

insurgencies. See "Congo's President Clings to Power," Editorial/Letters, *New York Times* (December 23, 2016): A22.

[4] The translation from French is mine.

In the days that followed the election, I also received a series of collective communications sent by the presidents, chancellors, provosts and deans to the faculty, students, staff and alumni of colleges and universities with which I have been associated. The initial ones, like the statement addressed to the University of Pennsylvania "community" (where I am an emerita professor), characterized the presidential campaign as "one of the most bitter, divisive, and hurtful in American history," and anticipated that "whoever won, millions of people [would be] terribly troubled by the results." In similar language, these statements expressed the hope that the ideals that the academic community "holds dear—inclusion, civic engagement, and constructive dialogue—will guide our nation's new administration, and that they will work hard to ensure opportunity, peace, prosperity for every group and every person that together form the diverse mosaic of the United States." In addition, these communications called attention to the fact that it was "a stressful time" for students and that on-campus resources were available to provide them with the support they might need.[5]

The next group of communications from heads of academic institutions that I received concerned alarming postelection racist incidents that had occurred in some university contexts. At the University of Pennsylvania, for example, black freshmen students were assailed by racist messages and images from a GroupMe account based in Oklahoma. Penn's president, provost and executive vice president responded with a statement addressed to the entire university community in which they declared that they were "absolutely appalled" by this "totally repugnant" account." "Our police and information security staff are trying to locate the exact source," they continued, "and to determine if any steps can be taken to block the account":

> We must reiterate how absolutely essential it is to the core values of our community, and also to the well-being of our society and world, that all persons be treated with the dignity and respect they deserve. The racism of this GroupMe account is profoundly inimical to what we stand for as a university. We will take every step possible to counteract its appalling bias. And we all stand together in solidarity with our Black students who have been so terribly targeted.[6]

In the third week of November, two weeks after the election, the presidents of the so-called Seven Sisters colleges—Barnard, Bryn Mawr, Mount Holyoke,

---

[5] "Statement to the Penn Community," November 9, 2016.
[6] "A Message to the Penn Community from President Amy Guttmann, Provost Vincent Price and Executive Vice President Craig Carnaroli Regarding Racist Messages to Penn Students," November 11, 2016.

Radcliffe, Smith, Vassar and Wellesley[7]—issued a public letter to Stephen Bannon, President-elect Donald Trump's choice as chief White House strategist and senior counselor. As a woman who is an undergraduate alumna of Smith, who is the recipient of a PhD from Radcliffe countersigned by the president of Harvard,[8] and who was a member of the Barnard faculty from 1955 to 1966, I had both a personal and professional interest in receiving this collaborative letter that was written in response to what Bannon had said about these institutions.

The letter referred to a "widely reported" 2011 interview with Bannon conducted by Political Vindication Radio, in which he "disparaged lesbians, feminists and alumnae of the historic Seven Sisters Colleges, all in one statement that we deliberately choose not to repeat here."[9] "Other reported comments by you reflect other forms of bias, including racism, anti-Semitism, and more," the letter went on to say:

> As the leaders of the Seven Sisters Colleges, we take deep exception to these comments and ask that you take a more expansive, informed and tolerant world view in your leadership role.
>
> We are proud of our alumnae and students, who represent the spectrum of sexual orientation, race, class and religion as well as political party. Our alumnae are accomplished leaders in all spheres of public and professional life; they are committed to their work, their families and their countries. Now, more than ever, we look to those who would lead the United States of America for a message of inclusion, respect and unity.

Toward the end of November, I received emails about the Deferred Action for The Childhood Arrivals (DACA) program from the presidents of some of

---

[7] Originally the Seven Sisters were women's colleges. However, on October 1, 1999, the Radcliffe Institute for Independent Study, which was founded in 1961 by the president of Radcliffe College, officially merged with Harvard University, thereby establishing the Radcliffe Institute for Advanced Study at Harvard University. And Vassar College became coeducational in 1969.

[8] In 1954, when I was awarded my PhD, this was the only form in which Harvard University granted PhDs to women. It was not until 1963, when Radcliffe's graduate school merged with Harvard's, that Harvard degrees were awarded to women for the first time.

[9] The statement that the heads of these schools chose not to repeat—because they wanted their letter to Bannon to be written in a respectful tone "to model the kind of discourse we hope to see from him"—was the following: "a bunch of dykes [...] from the Seven Sisters schools up in New England." He applied the disparaging term "dykes" to women of liberal, progressive political orientation as well as to women of lesbian sexual orientation.

the colleges and universities with which I have had relations over the course of my academic career. These messages emanated from what were by then more than 440 US institutions of higher learning that were collectively committing themselves to support this program, which was established by the executive order of President Barack Obama in 2012 to shield what are now estimated to be the 2.12 million teenagers and young adults—the so-called Dreamers—who came to the United States illegally as the children of immigrants. Under this program, qualifying individuals[10] register with the government for what is known as "deferred action," which provides recipients with two-year renewable protection against deportation, along with work permits and Social Security numbers.

It was in response to Donald Trump's campaign declarations about his intention to deport unauthorized immigrants, including immediately overturning DACA, and their concern about the effect that this action could have on the undocumented students enrolled in their institutions, that so many college and university presidents endorsed, signed and publicly issued statements in which they expressed their commitment to the renewal and extension of DACA, and to doing all they can to ensure the continued safety and success of the undocumented students on their campuses.[11] Their statements include testimonies to the ways in which the academic community currently benefits from these students' presence on their campuses, to the vital contributions that they expect them to make to the country in the future, and to the fundamental American values of equal access to education and equal protection under the law, regardless of nationality or citizenship status, that protecting, supporting and advocating for undocumented students constitutes.

I consider the stand that these schools have taken with regard to the "Dreamers" to be both admirable and reassuring.

* * *

On Friday, January 20, 2017, Donald J. Trump became the 45th president of the United States. I watched the entire ceremony on television. I was shocked by the content and tone of his inaugural address: by the apocalyptically dark

---

[10] One of these qualifications is that such young persons have not been convicted of a felony or major misdemeanor.

[11] Some of the colleges and universities have pledged not to allow Immigration and Customs Enforcement, Customs and Border Protection and US Citizenship and Immigration Services on their campuses unless required by warrant, and not to share any information about any undocumented student with these agencies unless presented with a valid legal process.

vision of American society that it set forth, by its belligerent chauvinism, pugilistic populism and nationalistic isolationism, by its vainglory, and by the meanness of its disrespect for the accomplishments of the three former American presidents who were seated on the inauguration platform.

Trump's speech was devoid of any allusion to what has been integral to every presidential inaugural address throughout American history: an eloquent expression of and fervid commitment to what sociologist Robert Bellah termed the American "civil religion": "the subordination of the American nation to the ethical principles that transcend it in terms of which it should be judged"—to the values and the rule of law embodied in the Constitution, and to a nondenominational God.[12]

"For too long," Trump declared, "a small group in our nation's capital has reaped the rewards of government while the people have borne the cost":

> Washington flourished, but the people did not share in its wealth. Politicians prospered but the jobs left and the factories closed. The establishment protected itself, but not the citizens of our country. Their victories have not yet been your victories. Their triumphs have not been your triumphs. And while they celebrated in our nation's capital, there was little to celebrate for struggling families all across the land.

He went on to describe what he contended was the "different reality" for "far too many of our citizens":

> Mothers and children trapped in poverty in our inner cities; rusted out factories scattered like tombstones across the landscape of our nation; an educational system flush with cash, but which leaves our young and beautiful students deprived of all knowledge; and the crime and the gangs and the drugs that have stolen too many lives and robbed our country of so much unrealized potential.

"This American carnage stops right here and stops right now," he exclaimed. What is more, he contended, "For many decades, we've enriched foreign industry at the expense of American industry, subsidized the armies of other countries, while allowing for the very sad depletion of our military. We've defended other nation's borders while refusing to defend our own." But "from

---

[12] Robert N. Bellah, "Religion in America," *Daedalus* 95, no. 1 (Winter 1962): 1–21, and Bellah's introduction to a reprint of this essay in Robert N. Bellah, *Beyond Belief: Essays on Religion in a Post-Traditional World* (Berkeley: University of California Press, 1991), p. 168.

this day forward," he proclaimed, "a new vision will govern our land. [...] It's going to be only America first. America first." Trump chose "America first" as one of his rallying cries, but it is unclear whether he had knowledge of the slogan's clouded historical relationship to a group that resisted America's entry into World War II before Pearl Harbor, and the anti-Semitism that became associated with it.

* * *

Following the inauguration, I received a copious flow of messages about the implications of Trump's becoming president. One of the most notable of these was an email from a friend regarding the White House website. "If you have not yet done so," he wrote, "spending some time on the new White House Web Site is informative, particularly in terms of what has been removed—all content related to civil rights, climate change, immigration, health care and LGBT issues."

Another was the text of the sermon a colleague who is an Episcopal priest delivered to his congregation on January 22, 2017. "Christianity is more than pious platitudes about patience and acceptance and maintaining an attitude of submission and letting things be what they are, even if they are unjust, unfair, and unreasonable," he had preached:

> In this past week when we remembered Martin Luther King, Jr., and inaugurated the 45th president of the United States, and witnessed massive demonstrations, we have to remember what Dr. King said: that we need "to be saved from that patience that makes us patient with anything less than freedom and justice."

He ended his sermon by quoting a prayer that the United Methodist bishop and theologian Will Willimon had offered up on Martin Luther King Jr. Day:

> Lord, forgive the sin of our patience. Anoint us with a fresh spirit of impatience, that we might be half as angry over political injustice and human meanness as you are, and that, in our impatience, we might be given the guts to do something about it.

* * *

The "massive demonstrations" to which the Episcopal priest referred were the Women's Marches that took place on January 21—the day after the inauguration. It is estimated that as many as three million persons in more than five hundred American cities of all 50 states participated in the marches. In addition, sympathy rallies and solidarity marches took place in some sixty other countries, among them Antarctica, Australia, France, Germany, Greece, Hungary, India, Lebanon, Mexico, Myanmar, New Zealand, Poland, Portugal, Serbia and the United Kingdom. Men and women marched in these demonstrations, which were multigenerational, as well. Their participants included children, young adults, middle-aged and elderly persons, and parents, grandparents and their progeny. The "women's rights are human rights" core message of the marches encompassed reproductive rights, equal pay, affordable health care, action on climate change and a "build bridges, not walls" perspective on immigrants and refugees. Especially the marches that took place in the United States were characterized by a strong protest against Donald Trump, his outlook, the policies he had espoused in his presidential campaign, and his behavior. This protest was symbolically expressed by the pink crocheted and knitted hats festooned with little cat ears which were worn by many of the marchers. They were called "pussy hats," in reference to a 2005 video recording in which Trump was seen and heard making vulgarly disrespectful remarks about how men with his attractiveness and power could grab women by their "pussy" and "do anything" with them.

Although I was not physically able to take part in any of the marches, I did so vicariously through relatives, friends, colleagues, students whom I am currently mentoring, and former students who participated and shared their experiences with me.

"We are planning to 'Rise Up' on the day after the inauguration at the women's marches," a once-student of mine wrote to me: "My children [...] are flying in for it. I plan to have a big group—[my wife] and me, our kids, my sister and her family. I think we all are going to have to stay vigilant and vigorous."

"It was certainly an incredible day!" a grandnephew who marched in Washington, DC, with his girlfriend exclaimed in an email to me. "There was so much resolve and energy in the masses. I know it's going to be a tough four years, but this should give us some hope."

From a professor of sociology with whom I have done collaborative research and coauthored publications, and who I taught when she was a graduate student, came an account of her march in Boston with her husband and small daughter. It was "especially uplifting," she said, that "as we marched, the residents in adjacent buildings would signal their support. We even got cheered by the municipal workers sitting atop of garbage trucks that were used to mark the route of the march." Her daughter, "in particular," she reported, "found it all terrifically exciting, and a good way to spend the first day of a terrible presidency." Her message was accompanied by a series of photographs that she said would make it possible for me to "take a virtual march" with them. She, however, hoped that I was "managing to stay calm and not allowing this to distract [me] from writing. We need your voice and wisdom more than ever," she generously concluded.

An older friend who has played an important part in editing several of my books sent me an email headed "Hello from the train!" as she was passing through Philadelphia with two friends, en route from Boston to the Washington, DC, march. She described "the mood in the Boston station and on the train [as] one of determined outrage." The friends accompanying her, she told me, were both writers. One of them was 83 years old and the other 77, like herself. "We don't know how arduous this adventure will be for us," she acknowledged, "but we can't imagine not doing it."

* * *

The process of writing this essay has heightened my awareness that I do not personally know anyone who voted for Trump, or who was not apprehensive about the actions that he and his administration may take. I do not regard this as a virtue. Rather, I consider it to be an indicator of my insulated ignorance about the sizeable number of Americans who supported Trump, their reasons for doing so, and the "Make America Great Again" positive expectations they have of him.

If I were still engaged in classroom teaching and the students enrolled in my courses expressed the desire to discuss with me and each other the social and cultural significance of the dynamics and outcome of the election, I would be responsive to their wishes. But I would make clear to them the ways in which I lack the relevant knowledge and understanding—especially regarding why so many white working-class persons who voted for Trump seem to believe that he has the empathic motivation and the knowledgeable competence to deliver them from their bleak economic situation and what they feel is their loss of relative status. I would also make it known to students that in common with the majority of academic social scientists, I am a "liberal" and a Democrat, who voted for Hillary Clinton. Upholding my commitment to standing up against bigotry of any kind, I would insist that our conversation proceed civilly, without stereotyping or caricaturing those who think differently than we do. I agree with journalist Nicholas Kristof that there is a danger of many of our colleges and universities becoming liberal "echo chambers," and that, as he wryly put it, "When students inhabit liberal bubbles, they're not learning much about their own country. To be fully educated, students should encounter not only Plato, but also Republicans."[13] Like Kristof, I think that it is "shortsighted to direct liberal fury at the entire mass of Trump voters, a complicated (and, yes, diverse) group of 63 million people": "Go ahead and denounce Trump's lies and bigotry," Kristof urges:

> Stand firm against his disastrous policies. But please don't practice his trick of "otherizing" people into stick-figure caricatures, slurring vast groups as hopeless bigots. We're all complicated, and stereotypes are not helpful—including when they're of Trump supporters.[14]

---

[13] Nicholas Kristof, "The Dangers of Echo Chambers on Campus," *New York Times*, December 10, 2016. www.nytimes.com/2016/12/10/opinion/sunday/the-dangers-of-echo-chambers-on-campus.html.

[14] Nicholas Kristof, "Trump Voters Are Not the Enemy." *New York Times*, February 23, 2017. www.nytimes.com/2017/02/23/opinion/even-if-trump-is-the-enemy-his-voters-arent.html.

Chapter 15

DONALD TRUMP'S EXECUTIVE ORDERS ON IMMIGRATION

On January 27, 2017, at 4:42 p.m., after only seven days in office, President Donald Trump issued executive order 13769 effectively banning nationals of seven countries (Syria, Iran, Iraq, Libya, Somalia, Sudan and Yemen) from entering the United States for the ensuing 90 days. The people who live in these countries are predominantly Muslim. The order, in addition, suspended the entry of refugees into the United States for 120 days and barred Syrian refugees from entering the country for an indefinite period. Until lawyers from the American Civil Liberties Union and several district court judges swiftly intervened, the order included provisions for the detention of persons legally authorized to live and work in the United States permanently—holders of so-called green cards.[1] Even though none of the acts of terrorism in the United States have been perpetrated by persons originating from these countries, the rationale given for Trump's executive order was "to protect" American citizens from "foreign nationals who intend to commit terrorist attacks in the United States; and to prevent the admission of foreign nationals who intend to exploit United States immigration laws for malevolent purposes."[2]

Partly because of the precipitous manner in which this order was issued, major domestic and international airports experienced chaotic disarray as security personnel implemented the new rules. This situation enhanced the great anxiety experienced by passengers from backgrounds associated with the order who were debarking from planes and by those awaiting their arrival in airport terminals. Under these circumstances and in this atmosphere,

---

[1] The United States Permanent Resident Card—an identification card that attests to the immigration status of a person authorized to live and work permanently in the United States—is known as a "green card" because green ink dominates the printing on the card. For permanent residents it is valid for 10 years and for conditional permanent residents for two years, after which time the card must be renewed.

[2] "Executive Order: Protecting the Nation from Foreign Terrorist Entry into the United States." www.whitehouse.gov/the-press-office/2017/01/27/executive-order-protecting-nation-foreign-terrorist-entry-united-states.

according to a spokesman for the US State Department, almost sixty thousand visas were revoked.[3]

Airport populations swelled with protestors, lawyers and others who arrived to support the arriving passengers and their families. Mobilized by social media and word of mouth, protest demonstrations by thousands of sign-bearing persons erupted in airports in Boston, New York, Washington, DC, Chicago, Dallas, Denver, Los Angeles, San Francisco, Seattle and elsewhere within a few hours after the order was issued. In addition, hundreds of civil rights and immigration lawyers and law students worked in airports around the clock to aid the detainees, including filing lawsuits on their behalf in several states.

Over the weeks that followed, a continuous wave of protests against the order was sustained by a wide gamut of civil rights and humanitarian organizations; leaders of institutions of higher education; physicians associated with medical schools, schools of public health and teaching hospitals; and spokespersons for communities of scientists, religious groups, industrial companies and cultural institutions. For example:

- The American Civil Liberties Union requested a temporary injunction to "block the deportation of all people stranded in US airports under Trump's new Muslim ban" and in this connection raised an unprecedented $24.1 million in one weekend.
- Around January 22, Doctors Without Borders/Médecins Sans Frontières (MSF) issued a public statement in response to Trump's executive order:

  With upwards of 60 percent of MSF's annual budget being spent on assistance to people forcibly displaced from their homes, and with our teams witnessing borders being closed to many of our patients trying to flee conflicts in Syria, Somalia, and elsewhere, these are core issues for the communities and people our teams serve every day.

  The executive order's indefinite ban on Syrian refugees is particularly harmful for millions of Syrians displaced by horrific violence. Nearly five million people have fled Syria into neighboring countries, including Jordan and Lebanon, which have populations smaller than many American states (the United States, by contrast, has accepted fewer

---

[3] Rachel Weiner, Justin Jouvenal and Ann E. Marimow, "Justice Dept. Lawyer Says 100,000 Visas Revoked under Travel Ban; State Dept. Says about 60,000," *Washington Post*, February 3, 2017. www.washingtonpost.com/local/public-safety/government-reveals-over-100000-visas-revoked-due-to-travel-ban/2017/02/03/7d529eec-ea2c-11e6-b82f-687d6e6a3e7c_story.html?utm_term=.33fe8e9dec97.

than 20,000 Syrian refugees). [...] The president's executive order will effectively keep people trapped in war zones, directly endangering their lives. [...]

Even as we have had to denounce the executive [order ...] related to the suspension of the refugee resettlement, we will still engage with the Trump administration as part of our efforts to raise awareness of how US policy can positively and negatively affect the international response to humanitarian crises.[4]

- Rush Holt, chief executive officer of the American Association for the Advancement of Science (AAAS), wrote a lead editorial in the February 10, 2017, issue of *Science* in which he characterized Trump's immigration ban as a "jolt against the local scientific enterprise" and exhorted his colleagues to "act for science" in responding to it. "Although the ban may not be permanent," he said, "its effects are already being felt [...] in the world of science":

Some expected participants will not be attending this year's annual meeting in Boston of the AAAS. [...] I understand that a Sudanese scientist who is to be recognized for excellent work by women in developing countries will not be present for her award. Furthermore, the head of the World Academy of Sciences, also from Sudan, has cancelled his trip to Boston. There are an unknown number of other such cases. The denial of entry is a detriment for the individuals, and it is also an affront to science. To me, the very real damage to science outweighs the very thin claim of enhanced national security. [...]

In my experience, many scientists are hesitant to do anything beyond expressing general dissatisfaction. [...] Perhaps the greatest source of hesitation is the traditional scientist's unwillingness to venture beyond the comfort zone of the technical world she or he knows. To fight the immigration order would mean stepping into political terrain, a scientist would say; taking part in a public event to promote science could tarnish science or appear confrontational. Based on a long career in science, with a substantial interlude in elected office, I say that these are excuses for inaction. Taking action is the best course to take when science is threatened or when science can illuminate public issues.[5]

---

[4] Jason Cone, letter to supporters of MSF, February 2017.
[5] Rush Holt, "Act for Science," *Science* 335, no. 6325 (February 10, 2017): 551.

- The American Council on Education sent a letter signed by 598 American colleges and universities to Homeland Security Secretary John F. Kelly, stating that those institutions of higher education "took seriously the need for the United States to remain the destination of choice for the world's best and brightest students, faculty, and scholars," as well as "the need to safeguard our nation":

> International exchange is a core value and strength of American higher education. Moreover, our nation's welcoming stance to scholars and scientists has benefited the U.S. through goodwill and a long history of scientific and technological advances that have been essential to the economic growth our country has experienced for decades. When they return home they are ambassadors for American values.
>
> Our nation can only maintain its global scientific and economic leadership position if it encourages these talented people to come here to study and work. America is the greatest magnet for talented people around the world and it must remain so.[6]

- In Lafayette Square outside the White House, a mass organized by young Catholics to celebrate their solidarity with refugees and immigrants was held on January 30. It was attended by more than 500 persons. Several of the bishops in the US Catholic Church released statements in which they characterized Trump's refugee ban as "a dark moment in U.S. history," pledged solidarity with Muslim refugees, and called upon Catholics to support migrants. "Welcoming the stranger and those in flight is not one option among many in the Christian life," they said. "It is the very form of Christianity itself."[7]
- One hundred evangelical pastors and authors signed and took out a full-page *Washington Post* advertisement addressed to President Trump and Vice President Pence. It denounced Trump's refugee ban, stating, "As Christian pastors and leaders, we are deeply concerned by the recently announced moratorium on refugee resettlement. As Christians, we have a historic

---

[6] Susan Svrluga, "Nearly 600 Colleges Object to Trump's Travel Ban," *Washington Post*, February 3, 2017. www.washingtonpost.com/news/grade-point/wp/2017/02/03/nearly-600-colleges-object-to-trumps-travel-ban/?utm_term=.ccb1aad889b5.

[7] Teresa Donnellan, "550 Attend Mass outside White House in Solidarity with Refugees," *America: The Jesuit Review*, January 30, 2017. www.americamagazine.org/politics-society/2017/01/30/550-attend-mass-outside-white-house-solidarity-refugees. Michael J. O'Loughlin, "Responding to Trump's Ban, Top Catholic Bishops Pledge Solidarity with Muslim Refugees," *America: The Jesuit Review*, January 30, 2017.

call expressed over two thousand years, to serve the suffering. We cannot abandon this call now."[8]

- "In response to the executive order [...] on immigration and separately regarding refugees," 41 "Boston Jewish religious, philosophical, civic, and human service organizations [came] together to say that these actions—which are causing anxiety, pain, and anguish throughout immigrant communities and our nation—are unjust":

> We urge our elected and appointed officials at all levels of government to do everything in their legal authority to protect our foreign-born neighbors throughout the Commonwealth. We urge our community and others to join together to ensure that the United States does not close our doors to immigrants and refugees. We urge our government to maintain and expand a policy of responsible leadership for the protection and resettlement of refugee families, including in the United States, and including innocent civilians fleeing the horrors of Syria.

> The Torah warns against the wronging of a stranger (*Ger*) in thirty-six places. Rabbi Jonathan Sacks[9] takes note that "there is something striking about this almost endlessly iterated concern for the stranger—together with the historical reminder that "you yourselves were slaves in Egypt." Sacks goes on:

> *Why should you not hate the stranger?—asks the Torah. Because you once stood where he stands now. You know the heart of the stranger because you were once a stranger in the land of Egypt. If you are human, so is he. If he is less than human, so are you. ... I made you into the world's archetypal strangers so you could fight for the rights of strangers—for your own and those of others, wherever they are, whoever they are, whatever the color of their skin or the nature of their culture, because though they are not in your image—says God—they are nonetheless in Mine. There is only one reply strong enough to answer the question: Why should I not hate the stranger? Because the stranger is me." [...]*

> The approach to addressing these issues that as announced this past week is rooted in a rhetoric of fear and demonization and a policy that treats human beings around the world [...] as an enforcement problem.

---

www.americamagazine.org/politics-society/2017/01/30/responding-trumps-ban-top-catholic-bishops-pledge-solidarity-muslim.

[8] Daniel Burke, "100 Evangelical Leaders Sign Ad Denouncing Trump's Refugee Ban." www.cnn.com/2017/02/08/politics/evangelicals-ad-trump/index.html.

[9] Rabbi Lord Jonathan Sacks is a British rabbi, philosopher and scholar of Judaism who was the chief rabbi of the United Hebrew Congregation of the Commonwealth from 1991 to 2013.

We believe that these issues must be approached as a humanitarian matter, with commitment to the welfare and dignity of all peoples. […]

We reject any effort to shut our nation's doors to the most vulnerable. We recommit ourselves to the work of protecting and advancing the dignity of all human beings and to preventing suffering in this world.[10]

• On February 5, a total of 97 technology companies filed a "friend-of-the-Court" brief with the Ninth US Circuit Court of Appeals in San Francisco, arguing that Trump's executive order temporarily banning immigration from seven majority-Muslim countries and all refugees would "inflict significant harm on American business":

Highly skilled immigrants will be more interested in working abroad, in places where they and their colleagues can travel freely and with assurance that their immigration status will not suddenly be revoked. Multinational companies will have strong incentives […] to base operations outside the United States or to move or to hire employees and make investments abroad. […] Ultimately, American workers and the economy will suffer as a result.

The brief also paid tribute to the contributions that "inclusive immigration policies" have made to the American economy—citing the statistics that immigrants or their children have founded more than two hundred of the companies on the Fortune 500 list, and that since the year 2000, "more than one-third of all American Nobel prize winners in Chemistry, Medicine, and Physics have been immigrants."[11]

• On the night of February 2, 2017, New York's Museum of Modern Art expressed its strong protest against Trump's executive order by rehanging part of its permanent collection, replacing seven of its works by Western European artists (among them Cézanne, Matisse, Picasso and Picabia),

---

[10] "We Must Not Close Our Doors": Communal Joint Statement on Immigration and Refugees, *Jewish Community Relations Council*, January 30, 2017. www.jcrcboston.org/communal-joint-statement-on-immigration-and-refugees/.

[11] "Nearly 100 Tech Companies File an Amicus Brief Opposing the Ban," *Washington Post* 2017. https://apps.washingtonpost.com/g/documents/business/nearly-100-tech-companies-file-an-amicus-brief-opposing-the-ban/2322/; Bill Chappell, "Nearly 100 Tech Firms Ask Federal Court to Block Trump's Travel Ban," National Public Radio, February 6, 2017. www.npr.org/sections/thetwo-way/2017/02/06/513703440/nearly-100-tech-firms-ask-federal-court-to-block-trumps-travel-ban.

which had been on permanent display, with works by "artists such as the Sudanese painter Ibrahim el-Salahi, the Iraqi-born architect Zaha Hadid and the Los Angeles–based Iranian video artist Tala Madani." Alongside each of these works the Museum placed a wall text that read:

> This work is from an artist from a nation whose citizens are being denied entry into the United States, according to a presidential executive order issued on Jan. 27, 2017. This is one of several such artworks from the Museum's collection installed throughout the fifth-floor galleries to affirm the ideals of welcome and freedom as vital to this Museum as they are to the United States.[12]

- And the Delacorte Public Theater in New York's Central Park announced that it would open its annual free Shakespeare in the Park productions in May with Shakespeare's *Julius Caesar*, described by journalist Maureen Dowd as a play "about a populist seeking absolute power." The theater said that the play had "never felt more contemporary."[13]

* * *

No one in my personal or professional networks is a citizen of a country listed on the Trump travel ban, or a current refugee. But virtually everyone with whom I am connected is deeply concerned about the origins, intentions and consequences of Trump's executive order. Among them are a number of persons—all of whom are former students of mine or mentees—who have reasons to feel especially strongly about its objectionable and harmful implications.

Vasanta Karunakara,[14] a sociologist who has an adjunct faculty appointment at a university in Philadelphia, confided to me in the course of a long telephone conversation that since Trump issued his order she has been "feeling like a foreigner" for the first time during the 15 years she has lived, studied and worked in the United States. Vasanta, who came to this country from India, has lawful, permanent residence here. But because she is "brown, rather than

---

[12] Jason Farago, "MoMA Protests Trump Entry Ban by Rehanging Work by Artists from Muslim Nations," *New York Times,* February 3, 2017. www.nytimes.com/2017/02/03/arts/design/moma-protests-trump-entry-ban-with-work-by-artists-from-muslim-nations.html?mcubz=0.

[13] Maureen Dowd, "Trump's Golden Lining," *New York Times,* February 11, 2017. www.nytimes.com/2017/02/11/opinion/sunday/trumps-gold-lining.html?mcubz=0.

[14] A pseudonym.

white," she told me, and some of her clothes "overlap in style" with those worn by Muslim women—although she does not wear a kerchief in the same way that they do—she now feels conspicuous in public spaces. For instance, when she goes shopping for groceries, even in what she considers to be the relatively cosmopolitan and safe environs of the university where she teaches, she finds herself taking extra precautions not to irritate the store's personnel by asking too many questions, or by seeming to be impatient when she is waiting in line for a cashier to tally up her purchases. Even though she has a green card that attests to her permanent residency status, and also has what she regards as "the best education in the world" that gives her what she considers the "advantage of the trained insight of a social scientist" into complex social situations, she still feels "vulnerable."

Samuel Heilman, a professor of sociology and holder of a chair of Jewish Studies at Queens College, CUNY (the City University of New York), was impelled to write a passionate article in protest against a president whose signature act is to close the door on refugees and build a wall to restrict immigrants. His article, "My Parents Were Saved on Schindler's List. Then America Took Us In," was published in the February 1, 2017, English-language edition of *Haaretz*, Israel's oldest daily newspaper. In this article Heilman recounted how, on Friday, January 13, 1950, along with another 1,295 displaced persons, his parents ("Holocaust survivors who had been on the now-famous Oskar Schindler's list)[15] and he, who was born in Germany after World War II and was three years old, arrived by ship in New York's harbor, docking at Pier 59 on West 19th Street in Manhattan. They were among "the lucky ones," he wrote, "designated to become permanent residents [of the United States] through the Displaced Persons Act, signed into law in June 1948 by President Truman. […] The number would eventually rise to 415,000." "Many of the refugees like us went on to build lives," he continued, "transforming a nation of immigrants into the true new colossus, the most powerful and free home of the brave, from sea to shining sea":

---

[15] Oskar Schindler (1908–1974) was a German industrialist, spy and member of the Nazi Party who saved the lives of 1,200 Jews during the Holocaust by employing them in his factory, originally located in occupied Poland and the Protectorate of Bohemia and Moravia. He convinced the commander of the nearby Kraków-Polaszów concentration camp to allow him to move his factory, and the 1,200 Jews who worked for him, to Brünlitz in Sudetenland. Their names were typed on a list that he submitted to SS officials, whom he continued to bribe to prevent the Jewish workers' incarceration in a concentration camp. In 1963 he was named "Righteous Among the Nations" by the Israeli government. Although he died in Germany, he was buried on Mount Zion in Jerusalem, "the only member of the Nazi Party to be honored in this way" ("Oskar Schindler," *Wikipedia, the free encyclopedia*, https://en.wikipedia.org/wiki/Oskar_Schindler).

As I grew into the social scientist and educator I now am, I understood through my own life experience and the facts on the ground that the decisions lawmakers and leaders of America had made to open their borders to immigrants—to people willing to take the risk of starting their lives over, learn a new language and reassemble themselves—were the true secret of America's continuing ability to revive itself and beat all challenges to its dominance. [...]

Mediocrities generally shun the competition of new challenges and seek to restrict immigration. A president who claims his goal is to "Make America Great Again," but whose signature act becomes to close the door on refugees, build a wall to restrict immigrants, and warns the rest of us to shut up if we protest this is dooming his nation to mediocrity.

And those who encourage or endorse such actions [...] are no better.[16]

Robert Klitzman, professor of psychiatry and director of the Master of Bioethics Program at the College of Physicians and Surgeons of Columbia University, sent an indignant letter to the editor of the *New York Times* regarding the paper's report, in a front-page story on January 29, 2017, bearing the headline "Ban Prompts Deep Anger, Muted Praise," that "some relatives of Americans killed in terrorist attacks said it was right on target." "As a family member of a victim of the 9/11 terrorist attack on the World Trade Center—my sister was killed—I am deeply offended," Klitzman wrote:

Mr. Trump's blunt order leaves thousands of innocent civilians stranded and aids terrorists who wish to portray the United States as anti-Muslim. Moreover, 15 of the 19 hijackers on 9/11 were from Saudi Arabia—excluded from Mr. Trump's list!

Over the past 16 years, over 100 times more Americans have been killed or injured by gun violence in the United States than were killed by terrorism, including 9/11.

Mr. Trump can make America safer through other, more thoughtful means, working closely with our Islamic and other allies, and reducing access to firearms.[17]

---

[16] www.haaretz.com/opinion/.premium-1.768811?=&ts=1486658.

[17] Robert Klitzman's letter to the editor was published along with several other letters, on January 29, 2017, on the Opinion Page of the *New York Times*, under the heading "The Outcry Over Trump's Refugee Ban." www.nytimes.com/2017/01/29/opinion/the-outcry-over-trumps-refugee-ban.html.

In her telephone and email exchanges with me following the proclamation of Trump's immigration and travel ban, Deborah Frank, the professor of Child Health and Well-Being and director of the Grow Clinic for Children at the Boston University Medical Center, expressed great anxiety over the possibility that the ban might "shatter" the professional work to which she has dedicated her professional life. As a clinician she treats children with so-called Failure to Thrive (FTT) resulting from malnutrition associated with poverty, homelessness, illness and family stress, and as the founder and principal investigator of Children's Health Watch, she conducts policy-relevant research on the health of infants, toddlers and preschoolers with the goal of improving their nutrition, health and development. She explained to me that although most of the children for whom she cares were born in the United States, many of their mothers are immigrants, some of whom are "undocumented" (although she does not know, or inquire into, whether they are documented). Furthermore, a significant number of the members of her staff and consultants are now facing immigration problems or may be confronted with them in the near future. In addition, she is concerned about whether funding for the kind of medical care and research in which she is engaged will be jeopardized by the outlook and policies of Trump's presidency.

At the age of 68 she is presently working on an 80 percent schedule rather than a full-time schedule, she informed me. Although she has been thinking about when she might retire, under the circumstances that are emanating from Trump's presidency, she is reluctant to do so. The best thing, she believes, is to continue to actively care for and about the children for whom she has been a committed advocate, and to keep the best possible records of the work in which she and her colleagues are engaged, so they have not only current but also future clinical value.

* * *

I strongly share the feelings and convictions of these individuals and groups who have expressed indignation and alarm about the attitudes toward immigrants and refugees that underlie Trump's executive order, and the action to temporarily or indefinitely suspend immigration to the United States by persons from certain Muslim-majority countries that it would mandate. My reaction is rooted in the values and beliefs that are fundamental to my personal and professional life history. As I have written elsewhere,

> both my mother and my father were the children of parents who emigrated from Russia and Romania to the United States at the beginning of the twentieth century. They were part of the great wave of East European Jews fleeing from religious persecution, the pogroms

of the Czarist regime, and poverty, who journeyed to "America" in the crammed steerage holds of ocean liners, and entered this country, which they regarded as the "land of opportunity," through the portals of New York's Ellis Island.[18]

Irrespective of the limited economic means with which my parents began their lives, and the extent to which this circumstance curtailed the number of years they attended school before undertaking full-time employment, they became impressively self-educated and achieved upper middle-class status. They in turn transmitted to their three children—my brother, sister and me— esteem for the life of the mind, and for achievements based on education and diligent study. And although we were raised in a secularized Jewish home, the Talmudic enjoinder to "love our strangers" as well as those whose national, ethnic, social class and religious origins were the same as ours was conveyed to us, both implicitly and explicitly, by our parents.

I am keenly aware that if my grandparents had not migrated to the United States, or had been denied entry to it when they disembarked at Ellis Island, the life that I have known as an American, which has been smiled upon in so many important ways, would never have come to pass. I am profoundly and everlast- ingly grateful for this. And in the lyric words of the poem by Emma Lazarus that is engraved on a bronze plaque inside the pedestal of the Statue of Liberty, I welcome and wish comparable good fortune for the "tired" and the "poor," the "homeless" and the "tempest-tossed," and to the "huddled masses yearning to breathe free" who now wish to enter this land and become part of it.

* * *

On February 3, 2017, in response to a suit brought by the states of Washington and Minnesota, US District Judge James L. Robart of the Federal Court for the Western District of the State of Washington issued a temporary nationwide restraining order (TRO) to halt the enforcement of Trump's travel ban. The TRO challenged the travel ban's constitutionality and stated that it "adversely affect[ed] the States' residents in areas of employment, education, business, family relations, and freedom to travel," inflicting damaging "harm" "upon the operations and missions of their public universities and other institutions of higher learning, as well as injury to the States' operations, tax bases, and public funds."[19]

---

[18] Renée C. Fox, *In the Field*, p. 7.
[19] United States District Court Western District of Washington at Seattle, Case no. C17-0141JLR. Filed 02/03/17. http://documents.latimes.com/seattle-judges-order-immigration/.

Trump reacted to this ruling with a series of aggressively derisive and accusatory tweets:

The opinion of this so-called judge, which essentially takes law enforcement away from our country is ridiculous and will be overturned![20]

When a country is no longer able to say who can, and who cannot, come in & out, especially for reasons of safety and security—big trouble![21]

Just cannot believe a judge would put our country in such peril. If something happens, blame him and court system. People pouring in. Bad![22]

If the U.S. does not win this case as it obviously should, we can never have the security and safety to which we are entitled! Politics![23]

Procedurally, the White House responded to the suspension of Trump's order by having federal attorneys in the Department of Justice immediately file an emergency motion asking the United States Court of Appeals for the Ninth Circuit[24] to overrule Judge Robart's TRO on the grounds that the executive order was "a lawful exercise of the President's authority over the entry of aliens into the United States, and the admission of refugees," and that the district court had "erred" in issuing a "sweeping nationwide injunction."[25]

On February 9, 2017, a three-judge panel of the United States Court of Appeals for the Ninth Circuit in San Francisco rejected Trump's petition to reinstate his travel ban.[26] They did so on several grounds—stating that the

---

[20] February 4, 2017, 8:12 a.m.

[21] February 4, 2017, 7:59 a.m.

[22] February 5, 2017, 12:39 a.m. See Peter Baker, "Trump Clashes Early with Courts, Portending Years of Legal Battles," *New York Times*, February 5, 2017. www.nytimes.com/2017/02/05/us/politics/donald-trump-mike-pence-travel-ban-judge.html.

[23] February 8, 2017, 7:03 a.m.

[24] The Ninth Circuit, which represents the most geographically diverse district in the United States, covers most of the western United States and also Hawaii and Alaska.

[25] Ariane de Vogue, "9th Circuit Court of Appeals to hear challenge to Trump's Ban Tuesday." www.cnn.com/2017/02/06/politics/9th-circuit-court-of-appeals-trump-travel-ban/index.html.

[26] The three members of the panel were Judge Michelle T. Friedland, who was appointed by President Barack Obama; Judge William C. Canby Jr., appointed by President Jimmy Carter; and Judge Richard R. Clifton, appointed by President George W. Bush.

administration had produced "no evidence" that anyone from the seven countries on the banned list had committed terrorist acts in the United States; that Trump's order seemed to violate some of the "due process rights" of lawful permanent residents of this country, and of refugees; and that although the president and the executive branch of the national government were entitled to deference in matters pertaining to immigration and national security, this does not mean, as Trump implied, that "national security claims are *unreviewable*, even if these actions potentially contravene constitutional rights and protection." Rather, "it is beyond question that the federal judiciary retains the authority to adjudicate constitutional challenges to executive action." Although the court noted that the states challenging the executive order had identified numerous statements by Trump about "his intent to implement a 'Muslim ban,'" it stated that it would defer making a decision about religious discrimination. But it did direct the Secretary of State and the Secretary of Homeland Security to give priority to refugee claims made by persecuted members of religious minorities. The only part of Trump's executive order that the court ruling did not affect was capping the number of refugees to be admitted to the United States in 2017 at 50,000—thereby reducing the 110,000 cap put in place under President Barack Obama.[27]

Trump immediately responded on Twitter to the Court of Appeals ruling: "SEE YOU IN COURT, THE SECURITY OF OUR NATION IS AT STAKE!" Notwithstanding this at once swaggering and threatening remark, he made it known that he intended to rework and reissue his travel ban. But before he did so, he instructed the Department of Homeland Security to "take the shackles off" arresting and deporting undocumented immigrants by Immigration and Customs Enforcement and Border Control agents. Furthermore, in the course of his first address to Congress, on February 28, he stated that he was in favor of a "merit-based" immigration system, and he announced that he had ordered the Department of Homeland Security to create an office called "VOICE" ("Victims of Immigration Crime Engagement") that would publish a weekly list of the crimes committed by immigrants. In addition, among the honored guests he invited to attend his address, and whom he put on public display, were four persons he described as "very brave Americans [...] the government had failed" when a 17-year-old boy who was a member of their family was murdered by a person Trump characterized as an illegal immigrant gang member who had just been released from prison.

* * *

---

[27] Adam Liptak, "Court Refuses to Reinstate Travel Ban, Dealing Trump Another Legal Loss." www.nytimes.com/2017/02/09/us/politics/appeals-court-trump-travel-ban.html.

On March 6, 2017, Donald Trump issued executive order 13780, a revised version of his blocked January 27, 2017, executive order. He unveiled this new order (to go into effect on March 16) without the media fanfare he had orchestrated to accompany its first version, which he had signed at the Pentagon, in the presence of many reporters. The only visual that appeared in connection with the immigration order issuance this time was a photograph of Trump sitting alone at his desk in the White House Oval Office signing the order. The overarching stated rationale given for this second version of the order, as for the original one, was "to protect the Nation from terrorist activities by foreign terrorists admitted to the United States":

> The screening and vetting protocols and procedures associated with the visa-issuance process and the United States Refugee Admissions Program (USRAP) play a crucial role in detecting foreign nationals who may commit, aid, or support acts of terrorism and in preventing those individuals from entering the United States. It is therefore the policy of the United States to improve the screening and vetting protocols and procedures associated with the visa-issuance process and the USRAP.[28]

The new executive order differed from the initial one in several respects:

- It removed Iraq from the list of the seven countries originally subject to a 90-day ban on travelers on the grounds that Iraq's "close cooperative relationship between the United States and the democratically elected Iraq government, the strong United States diplomatic presence in Iraq, the significant presence of United States forces in Iraq, and Iraq's commitment to combat ISIS justify different treatment for Iraq."[29]
- It exempted from the travel ban people from the other six countries on the list who are permanent, green card–holder residents of the United States, or who have a valid American visa.
- It reversed an indefinite ban on refugees from Syria, instead instituting a 120-day freeze requiring review and renewal.
- And it changed the language of the original version of the ban which had offered preferential status to persecuted minorities in those Muslim-majority countries, because this provision was widely interpreted as favoring other religious groups over Muslims.

* * *

---

[28] "Trump Travel Ban: Read the Full Executive Order." http://www.cnn.com/2017/03/06/politics/trump-new-travel-ban-executive-order-full-text/index.html.
[29] Ibid.

I am neither a lawyer nor a prophet. But I predicted that, like its predecessor, this revised version of Trump's original travel ban would be challenged by the courts before it went into effect, because it still singled out countries that are predominantly Muslim, and because it responded to the plight of refugees by admitting only 50,000 refugees to the United States each year—less than half the number allowed under President Obama. I also anticipated that a continuing struggle would ensue around these issues and around the ban's constitutionality. And I foresaw that this controversy would be accentuated, dramatized and prolonged by a recurrent pattern in Trump's behavior that Columbia Professor of Law Tim Wu has termed the "media strategy of 'continual warfare'" that has characterized his presidency since he assumed office.[30]

For this reason, rather than continuing to chronicle the saga of Trump's travel bans in this essay, I ended it on March 8, 2017. I did so with a mixture of apprehension about the ultimate outcome of Trump's attempts to ban immigrant travel, and hope that the courts and the collective protests by various groups and institutions in American society would continue to be effective in blocking the travel ban's implementation.

In spite of my declaration that I would end this essay with the foregoing paragraph, I felt impelled, one week later, to add to this essay an account of what rapidly ensued after Trump presented a revised version of his original travel ban.

States that tend to vote Democratic and nonprofit groups that work with immigrants and refugees immediately went to court to combat the revised order on the grounds that it thinly veiled the ban on Muslim immigration that Trump had promised to enact during his presidential campaign. Late in the evening on March 15, 2017, Judge Derrick K. Watson of the Federal District Court in Hawaii responded by issuing a nationwide order that temporarily blocked the revised version of the ban. He was joined overnight by Judge Theodore D. Chuang of the Federal District Court in Maryland. They agreed, in the words of Judge Watson's 43-page ruling, that the "illogic of the Government's contentions is palpable":

> The notion that one can demonstrate animus toward any group of people only by targeting all of them at once is fundamentally flawed. […]

> Equally flawed is the notion that the Executive Order cannot be found to have targeted Islam because it applies to *all individuals* in the six referenced countries. It is undisputed, using the primary source upon which the Government itself relies, that these six countries have overwhelmingly Muslim populations that range from 90.7% to 99.8%. It

---

30 Tim Wu, "How Donald Trump Wins by Losing," *New York Times*, March 3, 2017. www.nytimes.com/2017/03/03/opinion/sunday/how-donald-trump-wins-by-losing.html.

would therefore be no paradigmatic leap to conclude that targeting these countries likewise targets Islam. Certainly, it would be inappropriate to conclude, as the Government does, that it does not. [...]

When considered alongside the constitutional injuries and harms discussed above, and the questionable evidence supporting the Government's national security motivations, the balance of equities and public interests justify granting the Plaintiffs' [request to block the new order].[31]

In connection with their rulings, both Judge Watson and Judge Chuang referred to specific statements that had been made by Trump "leading up to and contemporaneous with his signing of the Executive Order" as examples of the "religious animus" behind it—in particular his call, when he was a presidential candidate, for "a total and complete shutdown of Muslims entering the United States." "Simply because a decision maker made the statements during a campaign does not wipe them from judicial memory," Judge Chuang wrote.[32]

At a rally that Trump held in Nashville, Tennessee, on the night of March 15, in the presence of what was reported to be "nearly 10,000 cheering supporters," he engaged in "an angry diatribe against the travel ban ruling and the judge [Watson] who had issued it." Trump prefaced his remarks by saying that he had some "bad [...] sad news" to share with his audience, about which, he said, "I have to be nice, otherwise I'll get criticized for speaking poorly about our courts." But he proceeded to characterize the judge's ruling as "terrible," and to claim that "in the opinion of many," it constituted "an unprecedented judicial overreach" that "makes us look weak, which by the way we no longer are, believe me," he asserted. "We're going to fight this terrible ruling," he bellicosely declared, by taking "our case as far as it needs to go, including all the way up to the Supreme Court." What's more, he threatened, since he regretted having revised his initial order, "going all the way" might include "going back to the first one."[33]

*** * ***

---

[31] In the United States District Court for the District of Hawai'i, CV. no. 17-00050 DKKW-KSW. Filed 03/15/17. www.pacermonitor.com/view/P52F2SY/State_of_Hawaii_v_Trump__hidce-17-00050__0219.0.pdf. See Laura Jarrett, "Trump Admin to Appeal Travel Ban Rulings 'Soon.'" www.cnn.com/2017/03/15/politics/travel-ban-blocked/index.html.

[32] Adam Liptak, "Campaign Pledge of Muslim Ban Haunts the President in Court," *New York Times*, March 17, 2017, pp. A1 and A13.

[33] Jarrett, "Trump Admin to Appeal Travel Ban Rulings 'Soon'"; Laura Jarrett, "Federal Judge Blocks New Travel Ban; Trump Calls It 'Judicial Overreach.'" http://fox13now.com/2017/03/15/federal-judge-blocks-new-trump-travel-ban/; Laura Jarrett,

Although the courts continue to protect the fundamental American values and precepts of the US Constitution that Trump's successive travel bans violate, and the media (other than those of the extreme right and the alt-right) continue to bear protesting witness to violations of these values and precepts, Trump relentlessly defies them and all those who question and challenge him. As a US citizen, I feel morally obligated to attentively keep abreast of his utterances and actions in relation to the ban, and also to closely follow his deeply troubling stances with regard to numerous other vital issues, among them those associated with health care in American society and with the allocation of resources in our national budget. Doing so heightens my anxiety, and borders on becoming almost obsessive to a degree that journalist Roger Cohen has likened to the threat of having "the mind of the American president come to inhabit people's lives."[34]

It drove me to write this alarmed addendum to an already long essay. Now, because on September 24, 2017, six days before the US Supreme Court was scheduled to hear arguments on his travel ban, President Trump has issued a revised one, I feel compelled to respond to it with another addendum.

This latest travel ban, scheduled to go into effect on October 18, definitively bans entry to the United States of most citizens of seven countries: Iran, Libya, Syria, Yemen, Somalia, Chad and North Korea. In addition, certain citizens from Iraq and Venezuela will face restrictions and heightened scrutiny. The rationale given for this action is that it will "protect the safety and security of the American people" by targeting countries that are not meeting the new minimum standards for identifying and screening potential travelers, and sharing relevant information about them with US law enforcement agencies. Notable is the fact that, with the exceptions of North Korea and Venezuela, the list of countries to which this latest travel ban applies are Muslim-majority countries. Furthermore, the ban that is involved is now indefinitely permanent, rather than confined to the 90-day restriction that Trump's first version of the ban entailed.

"Trump's Words Come Back to Haunt in Court." http://www.cnn.com/2017/03/16/politics/trump-campaign-statements-federal-lawsuits/index.html; Alexander Burns, "2 Federal Judges Rule Against Trump's Latest Travel Ban." https://www.nytimes.com/2017/03/15/us/politics/trump-travel-ban.html; Alexander Burns, "Federal Judge Blocks New Ban on Travel to U.S.," *New York Times* (March 16, 2017): A1 and A11; Julie Hirschfeld Davis and Maggie Haberman, "In One Rocky Week, Trump's Self-Inflicted Chaos on Vivid Display," *New York Times,* March 18, 2017. https://www.nytimes.com/2017/03/18/us/politics/trump-controversies-chaos.html.

[34] Roger Cohen, "Christo Wraps Donald Trump," *New York Times,* March 17, 2017. www.nytimes.com/2017/03/17/opinion/christo-wraps-donald-trump.html.

On September 25, 2017, the Supreme Court canceled the oral arguments on Trump's travel ban that had been scheduled for October 10. "The court asked lawyers in the case to submit briefs by Oct. 5 discussing the effect of Mr. Trump's new proclamation [...] replacing his revised travel ban, which had been issued in March. [...] The justices asked parties to address 'whether, or to what extent, the proclamation' may render the case moot."[35]

This development leaves open the possibility that the court may never decide on the case—a potentiality that increases my already great concern.

---

[35] Michael D. Shear, Ron Nixon, Adam Liptak, "Supreme Court Cancels Hearing on Previous Trump Travel Ban," *New York Times*, September 25, 2017. www.nytimes.com/ 2017/09/25/us/politics/trump-travel-ban-supreme-court.html.

Part 5

ON BEING A TEACHER

Chapter 16

ON BEING A TEACHER

One of the founders of sociology in the United States, Charles Horton Cooley, declared that teaching "ought to be practiced in joy," and for me, teaching truly has been a lifelong joy.[1] Since I became an "emerita" professor my encounters with students rarely take place in an academic classroom, yet being a teacher continues to be core to my identity.

When I told Allen Glicksman, the sociologist who directs research and evaluation at the Philadelphia Corporation of Aging, that I was planning to write an essay about the nature and scope of my relationships in the eighth decade of my life, he replied by saying that "connectivity is not only beneficial to older adults"; it also gives older adults "the opportunity to continue to play vital roles in the lives of others, and […] to contribute to their communities. […] It is therefore a social, as well as an individual, benefit."

Allen is one of the vast number of people with whom I am in continual contact through postal and email correspondence, telephone calls, the exchange of publications, photographs and holiday and rites-of-passage gifts, and face-to-face visits. Prominent among those with whom I have "connectivity" are former students—women and men I have taught over the course of my long academic career. When he was studying for his doctorate in sociology at the University of Pennsylvania, Allen was one of these students.

* * *

A moving face-to-face visit was paid to me by a former student of Indian origins whom I had taught many years ago. She referred to me as her "first university teacher and mentor," her "dear first guru," and she had timed her visit to coincide with *Guru Purnima*, which is the festival celebrated by Hindus on the full moon day in the months of June and July to pay their respects to their teachers and express their gratitude to them.

---

[1] Charles Horton Cooley, *Life and the Student: Roadside Notes on Human Nature, Society, and Letters* (1927; reprinted with a new introduction by Jonathan B. Imber, New Brunswick, NJ: Transaction Publishers, 2015), p. 83.

An email message came from Jenny, a physician, whom I taught when she was an undergraduate at the University of Pennsylvania. She had completed her first year in the bioethics program at Columbia University to which she had been admitted with a supporting letter from me. She wrote to tell me how much she had enjoyed it, and how valuable she felt it was in "opening [her] eyes to ethical dilemmas in [her medical] work" and in "contemplating them."

Another email was sent by Joanne, who had been enrolled in the introductory course in sociology that I taught during the 1960s at Barnard College, from which she graduated in 1969—which was 50 years ago. She is now 74 years old. Her communication brought dolorous news about the deaths of her mother and husband. She told me she was looking at her husband's books, and "all the books on Moby Dick caught my eye—and so my thought turned to you and your wonderful ethnobiography, *In the Field*, with your tale of studying Melville's great work." She was referring to my autobiography, and to what I described in it as my experience as an undergraduate at Smith College studying *Moby Dick* with Newton Arvin in his course on nineteenth-century American writers.[2] "I so hope you are well and still learning and thriving," Joanne's email concluded.

I also heard from Diya. Our relationship originated when she was a graduate student at the University of Pennsylvania in the Department of Sociology, where I was one of her teachers and a director of her dissertation, which was based on her medical sociological field research in rural villages of India. In one email she wrote to tell me about a critical incident that had just taken place in the context of the ethnographic study of an urban American charter school that she was currently conducting. In another she thanked me for a series of articles about India published in *The Economist* that I had sent her, and then praised me—over-lavishly—for being, in her opinion, one of the "few truly intellectual souls whose interest goes beyond her immediate work."

The email I received from Nathan, a professor of sociology whom I taught during his graduate student years, was a copy of the communication he had sent to the executive director of MSF-USA, asking if she would permit the journal he edits to publish the text of the "Renée C. Fox Medicine, Culture and Society Lecture" that she had delivered at the University of Pennsylvania School of Medicine.[3] "Renée and I go back some forty years," he told her, "when I first appeared at Penn as a graduate student in sociology and found her courses on medicine, society, and culture to be formative in my career as

---

[2] Renée C. Fox, *In the Field*, pp. 64–65.

[3] The lecture, titled "Saving the World, or Saving One Life at a Time? Lessons My Career with Médecins Sans Frontières Has Taught Me," delivered by Sophie Delaunay on May 5, 2015, was the seventh such annual lecture.

a sociologist. I have studied the intersections between religion and medicine for most of my career, having most recently published [… a book about] the decline of moral authority in American medicine. Renée's presiding presence in that work cannot be underestimated," he generously stated.

In addition to a continual flow of messages and visits from former students, I receive a variety of gifts from them. They include the cookies that Christine, a plastic surgeon, bakes and sends me every Christmas from California. In greetings on a recent holiday I heard from four women who took courses with me when I was a very young junior faculty member at Barnard College. They must be in their late 60s or early 70s now. One of them, a physician I taught when she was a Radcliffe undergraduate, made a donation in my honor to the medical humanitarian organization Doctors Without Borders/Médecins Sans Frontières (MSF).

Among the other gifts that I recently received was the offer from Alice, a lawyer, regarding my access to online journals. She asked via email whether as an emeritus professor I had access to the University of Pennsylvania electronic library. "If you do have access and don't know how to access it," she continued, "I can teach you in less than half an hour on the telephone":

> It gives me pleasure to forward articles to you that are of interest to you. You used to tear out articles and send them to me when I was working on my dissertation, and I always relished receiving each article from you. It made me feel so grown up, professional and collegial! So I am only too glad to forward articles to you, so you can have as much access as you want and deserve.

I also receive cards and gifts from students on Mother's Day! One is a Barnard College alumna who writes to me as often as every few weeks from the small town in Minnesota where she lives. Once, when we had been out of touch for longer than usual, she sent me a message expressing concern about how she would know if something happened and I was "in the hospital, or were in need of any kind. I would want to rush to your side," she declared, "or do whatever I could to bring you comfort and cheer." Accompanying a bouquet of flowers one Mother's Day was a note from her that read "Dear Renée, I've always been grateful for your maternal presence in my life." Another gift, of candy, arrived with a note thanking me for having "nurtured multitudes of students."

And one book delivered in the mail was a newly published work by a physician for whom I was an advisor and mentor when he was doing postgraduate study and research in the Robert Wood Johnson Clinical Scholars Program at the University of Pennsylvania. He had dedicated the book "To the men and women who shared their experiences with me for this book, and to Renée C. Fox for her extraordinary guidance and inspiration."

* * *

Many of the once-students with whom I have contact have become physicians or nurses. Implicitly, and sometimes quite explicitly, they are inclined to caringly watch over my health, and how I am managing my daily rounds:

> As the years go by our bodies become more frail; for example, I am discovering muscles and joints that never complained before but are now beginning to moan and groan at me. I can see how much greater this is in your case, and I do worry about you sometimes. […] May Rab (my preferred name for the Creator as it connotes one who nurtures and sustains) continue to hold you in her palm and always keep your spirit strong.
>
> Take care of yourself my friend and, inshallah, we shall meet again.

* * *

A notable attribute of the messages that I receive from past students is how vividly they remember our often long-ago encounters. This surprises me, because I would have assumed that with the passage of time those memories would have dimmed. In some instances the student and I have maintained a continuous relationship, as is the case with Dana, who recently thanked me for a contribution I made to the pediatric and obstetric research institute she founded and directs. That gift's "meaning was all the more special," she wrote, "because it came from you, and you have given me so much wisdom over the past **40** years (my seminar with you was 40 years ago this spring!)." In other instances, triggered by a professional or personal event, former students from whom I have had no communication for many years will suddenly make contact with me:

> Subject: Dr. Fox: get your memory shoes on
>
> Dear Dr. Fox:
>
> You were my all-time favorite teacher while I attended Penn back in the eighties. […] I know that you cannot possibly remember me, given the thousands of students that you have touched, but this one has been touched again. You took me out to lunch and heartily laughed when I blew on my cold soup. […] Do you still live in your apartment in Rittenhouse Square?

Well anyway, if you get this message and would be so kind to mail me back, I would be extremely grateful. [...] You were kind to me and treated me like I hadn't been treated before, which I know you must have done to thousands of people, but your kindness still resonates thirty years later.

Here's to you, Dr. Fox. Thank you for just being there when you were.

Your student, your friend,

Roy

###

Subject: Thank you, from a former (very former) student

Hello Dr. Fox.

I would like to think you again for allowing me to take your very enlightening graduate seminar many years ago. It is one of the few courses from my undergraduate days that I do remember, and remember as being influential. I believe I thanked you then, since you kindly allowed me to take your graduate medical sociology seminar at Harvard, when I was a somewhat naive undergraduate, and just as I was beginning to consider a career in medicine. However, it seemed to me good to give you a second thank you, to let you know that the concepts your teaching inspired, more than many other aspects of my "soc. rel" [Social Relations] major, have stood the test of time, and been a very positive influence. I still have *Experiment Perilous*[4] on my bookshelf, and still find a sociological view of medicine fascinating and informative. [...]

I'm still in medicine, in Seattle, and do some teaching as well.

We often forget to thank people, and I'm not sure how I came to check in on your career at this point. Perhaps the thought occurred to me as I was suggesting to one of my daughters that she also thank a former professor. Perhaps seeing your MSF book,[5] which I am now reading.

###

Dear Renée:

I am sitting in a "mentoring" class. The instructor has asked us to write a note to a cherished mentor. Here goes. I am writing to thank you for

---

[4] Fox, *Experiment Perilous.*
[5] Fox, *Doctors Without Borders.*

making time to give me your attention, for making room in your thoughts to consider what I needed in my personal and professional development, for taking the steps that were needed to help advance my career, and for caring enough to share your wisdom about what is important in life. These gifts have made it possible for me to follow a very rewarding path in my life.

###

My dear teacher Dr. Fox,

Hope this email found you well. It is amazing how time flies, and it has been twenty-eight years since I graduated from Penn, and that was the last time I saw you.

Well, fast forward to now, my son is ready to start high school this fall and we plan to visit Philadelphia and Boston in June for his possible future college consideration. Our travel schedule will bring our family to Philadelphia on June 11 & 12. Our family would very much like to get together with you for lunch or dinner if those dates work for you. I look forward to hearing from you soon.

In this and many other instances my continuing contact with former students and my occasional contact with others involves their children. Laura, whom I taught when she was an undergraduate, lives in Philadelphia and makes periodic visits to my apartment with her sons, Jason and Kasper. We often spend some of our time together in Rittenhouse Square Park. For reasons neither of his parents nor I understand, Jason insists on using my full name—"Renée C. Fox"—when he speaks of me, or to me. He cannot be persuaded simply to call me "Renée." As soon as he and his younger brother Kasper arrive, they make an exuberant beeline for their favorite places in my apartment: to the kitchen, where I keep an aluminum "reacher" shaft with a magnetic tip that makes it easy to pick up objects without bending, which they enjoy playing with; to my study, where they are attracted to a ball-bearing paperweight on my desk, and where Jason clambers up into the desk chair and, using one of the pens and pads arrayed on the desktop, proudly prints his name. From the study, the two of them usually race to my bedroom. There they gaze with delighted wonder at the panoramic urban view they can see through the room's floor-to-ceiling windows. Mementos of their visits are affixed with magnets to my refrigerator door: a photo of Jason studiously writing at my desk, and one of Kasper smiling happily on a path in Rittenhouse Square Park.

One recent summer Jason attended a sleepaway camp for the first time. From camp he sent me the following letter, hand-printed in pencil:

Dear Renée C. Fox

I'm sorry I write so late; I just didn't have time to write earilyer [*sic*]. I'm having a lot of fun. When we went today [to an amusement park] I won a green bear. The way I won it is we had to shoot a water gun and hope that it makes your boat move. My boat got to the top first so I won.

Love,
Jason

* * *

A rather dramatic story underlies and antedates the connection I have with Nathaniel Kaufman, whose Bar Mitzvah I attended when he reached the age of 13. At the synagogue where this coming-of-age ritual took place, his father, Dr. Kenneth (Ken) Kaufman—who had in the late 1960s audited the sociology of medicine course that I taught when I was a lecturer at Harvard—arranged for me to have the honor of being one of the persons called to stand before the Holy Ark where the Torah scrolls are stored, at the point in the service when they were about to be removed from the ark for a relevant portion of them to be read by Nathaniel.

"I wonder how I could ever have been so lucky as to wander into your classroom," Ken once exclaimed in an email message. He was referring to how unlikely it had been for him to attend my medical sociology course, and to the disconsolate frame of mind in which he had done so. Ken, who was studying for a PhD in chemistry at the time, had just been told by his teachers in the Harvard Department of Chemistry that because he had epilepsy and was subject to the risk of recurrent seizures, it was too dangerous for him to do laboratory work with synthetic organic chemicals. His dream of being an organic chemist was thwarted.

He ultimately persuaded the chemistry faculty to permit him to pursue graduate studies in theoretical organic chemistry, in which he received a master's degree, after which he enrolled in medical school. At the time that he attended my medical sociology course he was still involved in the study of theoretical organic chemistry, which "paled compared to what I learned in your class," he once generously told me; the course also contributed to his decision to enroll in medical school. The contents of the course, how I taught it, and the way I "guided" him as his "pivotal mentor," he claims, "assisted [him] in becoming the person, clinician and academic that [he is] today":

My academic focus has been epilepsy, antiepileptic drugs, bipolar disorder, comorbid medical conditions, and social themes. […] I now have treated 34,000 patients. Their lives have impacted mine and have served to make me a more caring person. […]

Even my epilepsy […] has been a blessing, for it has forged a stronger, more committed soul to accomplish and to accept all. […]

My desire has [also] always been to be involved with students. […] [T]he process of both teaching and learning simultaneously has been one of my greatest joys. […]

I am ever mindful of your wisdom and can simply sit and read your books and articles to feel academically excited and at peace at the same time. […]

Further, in your writings and our correspondence, I have learned to appreciate life more fully, with a deeper satisfaction for what I have, what I can do, but not what might have been. […] I see you in my mind's eye every day and you always serve as a beacon of truth.

Recently Ken wrote me that he had just received notification of his election to Fellowship of the Royal College of Psychiatrists: "I wanted you to be one of the first to know that I am being honored for my career in psychiatry":

I am thrilled that [my wife] will be present to mark this special occasion. My mother would be especially proud. When thinking if there is anyone else I would want present (besides my children), I can only think of you, for you have been my lifelong mentor, have known me since the beginning days, and know so much about my life and career. I [know] that your attendance is not possible, but I wanted you to realize how significant you are to me.

The next piece of "exciting family news" that Ken shared with me via email concerned Nathaniel's 21st birthday and the job offer Nathaniel had just received from Microsoft, to begin upon his graduation from college. "To think of all that happened since you were my professor," Ken exclaimed, and then affirmed, in the conclusion of his message, "Your presence at Nathaniel's bar mitzvah will always be a special family memory." A short while later, Ken wrote to me again, this time accompanied by a photograph of his son:

Dear Renée,
Here is Nathaniel marching out after having been conferred his BS in Computer Engineering. A very special boy. A very special day.

We have shared many things over the years and having been such a large part of my life, I knew you would enjoy this photo.

Our bar mitzvah boy now starts an independent journey on his yellow brick road. May he always learn, search, and have lifelong mentors.

* * *

Events take place that give me the sense of being connected with an even larger number of former students than those from whom I have heard directly. I would have been unaware of the fact that Adele Clark, a prominent professor of sociology with recognized distinction in the field of medical sociology, whom I taught when she was a Barnard undergraduate, had made a gift in my honor to the college, if its executive director of individual gifting had not sent me a letter informing me of her contribution. When I wrote to Adele to thank her for her gift, she replied by saying, "I am the one honored by having you as my major sociology teacher undergrad, and it was a pleasure to give my little gift in your honor. I will do so again."

In 2015 Adele received the Reeder Award that is given annually by the American Sociological Association for "Distinguished Contribution to Medical Sociology [through] an extended trajectory of productivity that has contributed to theory and research" in the field, and for "teaching, mentoring, and training as well as service to the medical sociology community broadly defined." "I have meant to write to you since I received the Reeder Award," she emailed me. "I had a picture of you in my slide show as one of my most important teachers, with the year you won the Reeder. […] I attach a couple of photos from the events. The larger group is advisees of mine who were there that day. Sweet." It was clear from the joyous smile on her face in the photo with her advisees that what she considered to be the greatest honor that she had received on this occasion was the presence of the students whom she had taught, and the teacher-to-student chain that it represented of which we are both a part.

* * *

There is another group I am connected with in a kind of teacher-student relationship but whom I have never taught in a conventional way. They are individuals who have come to know me through my publications. My contact with Fred began when he introduced himself to me via email as a general internist and palliative care physician who was involved in outcomes research and evaluation in a medical center in Maine and who had a special interest in uncertainty in health care: "I've long been a great admirer of your pioneering work in medical uncertainty, which has influenced me greatly in my own thinking. I am writing to see if it was possible to talk with you by phone sometime to get your perspective and guidance on some research ideas and interests." I encouraged him to call, and in anticipation of our conversation he sent me several of his recent papers. Following these exchanges, he asked if I would provide him with "mentorship and guidance" for the book project he was working on, which I agreed to do. In 2015 and 2016 he made several trips to Philadelphia to meet with me in my apartment, where each time we talked for hours about his conception of the book concerning medical uncertainty that he is writing. "It was a real pleasure visiting and finally meeting you in person," Fred emailed after his first visit. "Our conversation yesterday gave me a fresh perspective on things. I left feeling very energetic and excited about doing more thinking and writing, and I really look forward to more conversations and work together!" Our relationship, via correspondence, face-to-face visits and the exchange of manuscripts, has continued and grown closer as the writing of his book has progressed.

There is also Ramanan in New Delhi, India, whom I have never met but for whom I became a tutor and dissertation advisor from afar after he initiated email contact with me. He wrote to me recently to say, "I have happy news to share": "I have submitted my PhD thesis successfully, and thanked you in my acknowledgements from my heart [for your] comments, suggestions and help."

* * *

These are some of the gifts of connectedness that over time and space I continue to receive from students—gifts that make being a teacher an ongoing source of energy, meaning and happiness for me. What is more, as one of my long-ago students generously testified, through this role I have been able to link some of those I have taught to a chain of teachers and mentors whose sense of vocation and vibrant heritage span past, present and future generations:

> Last night at dinner the conversation turned to teachers and mentors who changed our lives. Immediately your name came to mind. I told the story of how as a young Penn student I started taking classes in sociology and how you encouraged me and helped me to realize that I could actually think as a sociologist. […] You were a kind and generous teacher who met regularly with me as I embarked on graduate study and later wrote a dissertation. At each step, you challenged me to think with rigor and provided me with a role model for how to be a mentor. You even

introduced your students to your mentor and teacher, Professor Talcott Parsons, who we then experienced as a memorable teacher.

In the process you really changed my life and I have sought to emulate your ethical values, caring and scholarly conduct in my family life and career.

I want to say *thank you* and to give voice to how much gratitude I have for your guidance, support, and intellect.

* * *

My role as a teacher also seems to have played a part in the bonding of some of my former students to each other. An instance of this took place not long ago in Washington, DC, between two women physicians whom I taught when they were undergraduates. One, Nancy, had held an important public health position in the US Department of Health and Human Services for several years. The other, Deidra, held a directorship at the National Institutes of Health. Nancy appended a postscript about their meeting in Washington to the Christmas/New Year's greeting she sent me. "Had a wonderful reunion with Deidra this week," she wrote. "She brought me a copy of your memoir—but I had already read it! Will let you know when I come to Philly."

* * *

What I regard as the supreme teaching opportunity I have recently been given was accorded to me at the beginning of 2017. Its intermediary was Eric Ward, a medical student at the University of Pennsylvania who is an aspiring writer and a recognized poet. He was introduced to me by the author, journalist, editor and teacher of writing, Anne Fadiman, in whose nonfiction writing seminar at Yale he was a notable student before his admission to medical school.

The long email message that I received from him in January began with what he termed "a request": "Would you be willing to serve as the faculty adviser for the non-fiction writing group—called the "Gawannabes"—I am starting?"[6] This group of medical students, he went on to explain, "will be meeting at least twice a month in a formal workshop":

Half the time will be spent discussing a piece of writing by an established doctor-writer with an eye to its craft, and the other half will be devoted

---

[6] The group adopted this name because they consider the renowned surgeon-writer Atul Gawande to be a role model.

to reading and critically evaluating a piece of writing from one of the group's members. Additionally, we hope to have at least one visiting writer come per semester for a larger event, open to the entire medical school.

As the faculty adviser, your obligations to the group could be as large or as small as you wish. I could easily add you to our group email exchanges, where all work for revision (as well as any available electronic readings) will be exchanged. We would welcome any written feedback on the work that you might be willing to provide on the pieces we discuss, by students or otherwise. And as the group's leader, I would also be seeking your advice (in an additional capacity than I already do now!) or suggestions for readings, or possible speakers to invite. Your knowledge of the university as a whole, as well as your historical knowledge of how doctors and doctors-to-be have grappled with the experience of their training, would really be invaluable to us.

Eric was in the process of negotiating to make arrangements for the workshops to be held at the Kelly Writer's House,[7] he said, and he was hoping that larger events with outside speakers could be hosted at a time of the day, and a location easier for more people to attend.

I did not need the time to "think over" Eric's invitation. I was immediately excited and enthusiastic about it. It had come from an exceptionally intelligent and creative medical student and writer who held a strong commitment both to teaching and to learning and who was endowed with impressive organizational and leadership abilities. Furthermore, he was a protégé of Anne Fadiman, who has enriched my life through her role as an editor, the quality and message of her writing, and her colleagueship and friendship.[8] In

---

[7] Kelly Writers House, a 13-room house on the campus of the University of Pennsylvania, is a center for writers affiliated with the university and from the Philadelphia region more broadly. It was founded in 1995 by a group of Penn students, faculty and staff. The hundreds who visit the house each week write and collaborate in its seminar rooms and its publication office. And every academic semester, the house hosts as many as 150 public programs that include poetry readings, film screenings, radio broadcasts, art exhibits, musical performances, seminars and lectures.

[8] Among Anne's publications, the work that continues to have the strongest, most meaningful impact on me is her at once profoundly moving and deeply humane book *The Spirit Catches You and You Fall Down: A Hmong Child, Her American Doctors, and the Collison of Two Cultures*, a firsthand account of how the lack of cultural understanding between the physicians in a small hospital in California and a refugee family from Laos led to a tragic outcome for a Hmong child diagnosed with severe epilepsy, despite her having parents and doctors all of whom wanted what was best for her. From 1994 to 2000, under the aegis of Anne Fadiman's editorship of Phi Beta Kappa's journal, *The American Scholar*, I served as a member of its editorial board. Subsequently, it was through her

addition, it offered me the opportunity, as Eric put it, to "make connections with some of the other curious and creative individuals in [his] medical school class," and to draw on my many years of firsthand research on what being a physician and becoming a physician entail. The group's focus was also attuned to the literary, nonfiction, ethnographic writing that characterizes most of the books and articles I have published.

However, as I explained in my reply to Eric, I had a "major limitation" that he might "understandably feel would disqualify [me] to serve as the group's faculty adviser": "Although I am blessed with underlying good health, because of my age and the post-polio concomitants superimposed on my elderly body, I move about with the aid of a rolling walker":

> Whereas until recently I was able to navigate on my own with the walker, including taking taxis to locales outside my immediate neighborhood, it has now become perilous for me to do so without accompanying help. Therefore if your plan would be to meet regularly at the Kelly Writing House, the challenge would be for me to get there and back. [...] There would also be the question of how handicapped accessible that building is. And I would be very reluctant to ask someone in your group to fetch me each time there is a meeting and transport me back.

Alternatively, might the Gawannabes be a small enough group that they could meet in my apartment's study? Or, without my physically appearing at the planned locus of their meetings, was it possible that I could play an advisory role by suggesting some of the reading the group would do, reading and commenting on the manuscripts they would produce, proposing doctor-writers whom they might invite as speakers and connecting them with relevant persons on the Penn campus?

Without hesitancy or equivocation, Eric assured me by telephone that although I might not be able to physically attend the group's meetings, what I had described as the role I could play would fulfill all that they expected of a faculty adviser. This was followed by an email message from him informing me that the group's first meeting would probably not be scheduled before his medical school class's first graded exam. He would "touch base" with me by phone sometime around then, he said, so he could share some of his

---

intermediary that the extraordinary editor William Whitworth agreed to edit my auto-biography, *In the Field*. A fuller account of my relationship to Anne Fadiman, including the trip that we made together to visit Bill Whitworth in his hometown in Little Rock, Arkansas, appears in Renée C. Fox, "'Dear Mr. Whitworth/Dear Professor Fox': Ode to an Editor and Editing," *Society* 48, no. 2 (March/April 2011): 102–11.

ideas about the group and hear some of mine. "I'm so happy to have you on board," he concluded.

I sent an account of these exchanges with Eric to Anne Fadiman, thanking her for having introduced him to me in the way that she had, telling her how pleased I was to be invited to become the faculty adviser to the medical students' writing group that Eric was launching at Penn, and expressing my gratitude for the generosity he had shown in assuring me that I could serve in this capacity despite the limitations in my mobility. "Eric wrote me about the Gawannabes," she replied, "and about his hopes that you would be the adviser. […] I'm so glad that you can be […] (lucky Gawannabes!) and that you don't have to attend the meetings":

> I do hope that with Eric's help you can get to one meeting in 2017, or maybe have it in your apartment, so that the members of the group can have the pleasure of meeting you.
>
> It pleases me NO END that you and Eric have become such good friends.

This is how it has come to pass that, notwithstanding my age and my limited mobility, I have been given a privileged and uplifting new way to be a teacher.

* * *

In Memoriam

This essay is dedicated to Melissa Anne Goldstein, a student who became my intimate and cherished friend and colleague. She died at the age of 46 while I was in the early stage of writing this essay. The cause of her death was the autoimmune disease lupus—that Melissa often referred to as "the wolf"—with which she was diagnosed in the late 1980s, toward the end of her freshman year at the University of Pennsylvania.[9] During a period in her sophomore year, when she took a temporary medical leave from her college studies, Melissa made contact with me through correspondence. Our

---

[9] "Lupus" is the abbreviated term that is used to refer to the chronic inflammatory disease *systemic lupus erythematosus*, which occurs when the body's immune system attacks its own tissues and organs. It has the potential of affecting many different parts of the body, including the joints, skin, kidneys, blood cells, brain, heart and lungs. Lupus is also the Latin word for *wolf*. Historians seem to be unsure whether the name originally referred to a disease or to an injury that resulted in the destruction of surrounding tissue. But there appears to be speculative consensus that the name lupus has some relationship to the destructive injuries that can result from the bites of an animal like a wolf.

exchanges developed into an ongoing discussion of matters concerning medicine, literature, and the relationship between them. As I wrote to her mother:

> From the outset of my coming to know Melissa, her gift as a writer—especially as a poet—her exceptional intelligence, insight, and self-knowledge, her effervescence, and her valor were apparent to me. We bonded through our correspondence, and when she returned to Penn, somehow it seemed perfectly natural to me to invite her to co-design and co-teach with me a Freshman Seminar—"Medicine and Literature: The Physician Writer" (Sociology 041)—that we conducted together for several years. I think it was probably unprecedented for an undergraduate student to be cast in the role of a college faculty member.

That shared teaching experience strengthened and enriched our bond, to which my love of literature, the yearning writer within me, and the physical challenges I was experiencing due to the onset of post-polio symptoms in my aging body also contributed. My medical issues were minor compared to what Melissa was enduring as her lupus progressed, but with great generosity and empathy she saw connections between them.

Over the ensuing years we nourished and enjoyed our friendship and colleagueship, partly through periodic visits when she was living in an apartment in Center City, Philadelphia, and moving energetically about in her electric wheelchair. During this time she published her first book, *Travels with the Wolf: A Story of Chronic Illness*, which was based partly on the thesis she wrote for the master's degree she undertook at Penn after graduating magna cum laude from the college.[10] I had the honor of introducing her and her book to the gathering assembled for the reading she gave at the Penn Book Center in November 2000. What I said on that occasion was that Melissa not only had "the literary gifts, the profound perceptions, the sensitive insights, and the attunement to the human condition of a writer," but that writing was "her vocation—integral to her very being, and to the life's journey on which she is embarked." In addition, it was her "way of coping with the most challenging, arduous, and fearsome things that life [has asked] of her":

> Through the interweaving of her distinctive prose and poetry, she illuminates and transforms what might otherwise be unendurable or inexplicable into something that has positive, even uplifting meaning for

---

[10] Melissa Goldstein, *Travels with the Wolf: A Story of Chronic Illness* (Columbus: Ohio State University Press, 2000).

more than herself. And she does this without compromising veracity, or cosmetically removing the shadows and the dark places from the experiences of which she writes.

Later, when because of "the wolf's" ravages it was no longer possible for Melissa to live on her own, she returned home to her parents' house (evocatively located on a street named "Bittersweet Drive"). We maintained our correspondence, interspersed with occasional telephone conversations. The flow of her long, expressive, impeccably typed letters was sporadically interrupted by interludes of crisis in the trajectory of her illness. These included periods when because of her brain and spinal cord involvement she felt that her "mind was being lost or dulled in a lupus fog," and when troubles with serious infections, bleeding, cataracts and diabetes occurred that were largely attributable to the side effects of her lupus medications. At one point she underwent eight consecutive weeklong hospitalizations in the midst of which she wrote me a six-page letter penned in what she apologetically characterized as "inelegant [...] non-spell checked [...] beetle scratch handwriting."

Our exchanges, Melissa contended, "help me to retain my sense of myself as writer, as poet, during [...] difficult periods of ill health." And when she had what she referred to as "a tiny window" that enabled her to write a new poem, she enclosed a copy of it in her letter to me. ("Just a small offering. I would appreciate your opinion. [...] You have always done me the honor of being honest, and I would never want that to stop!")

Through it all, she continued to be what she called a "nutty optimist"—"a cup-half-full," rather than "a glass-half-empty person," who was also grateful for the ways in which she was "blessed":

> Whatever I have gone through, my situation could be worse. I could be alone in the world, like so many—and unable to afford even basic care. I have some truly wonderful health care professionals watching out for me. My friends and family nourish me with their love, their laughter, their inclusion of me in their lives. I deeply miss my life in Center City, but on the other hand, I've had a chance to know and spend time with my parents at a point in our lives when most parents and their children, in today's society, go their separate ways. [...] So with the loss of my independence, painful as it is, there is also some gain.

And in every communication that she had with me over time, she never failed to express her caring concern about *my* state of health, and a lively interest in my intellectual activities, especially my writing:

> I was glad to hear that your health remains relatively stable. I hope this letter finds this still to be true. I am happy to hear that you are able to

ask for the help you need, and thereby preserve as much independence as possible. It is an art, asking for and accepting help, as we have talked about over the years. […]

I am also thrilled to hear you are writing your book on Doctors Without Borders. It will be fascinating I am sure. I am not an expert on the literature published on DWB, but what I have read or seen in documentary form has not been very critical, only celebratory. A thorough analysis with your keen, insider viewpoint would really add to our understanding of the group, and groups like them—the forces which shape their creation and how they function.

The last letter that I received from Melissa was dated September 23, 2012. "My dearest friend," she wrote:

I am very sorry I disappeared during these past few months. As you probably guessed, the wolf and his attendants have been particularly vicious and constant. […] These "flares" were especially disturbing, […] involving organs and problems which have not troubled me before. It was as if my entire body underwent a storm in which the kidneys, liver, skin, endocrine system […] etc. all showed significant forms of attack.

I am spending my days in a consuming routine of medical care, something I swore I would never do. I am struggling to retain some part of every day as mine, even an hour which is unrelated to illness, and in that way keep that part of myself which is Melissa, free of illness, alive and flourishing. To change metaphors, it is like tending a tiny hidden patch of a lush flowering garden, an untouched place unlike the surrounding land so brown and bleached, blighted by the wars fought all around. […]

I hope we will find some treatment options soon which will allow me to expand my garden tending. But until then, I will do the best with what I have now, breathing deeply each day, knowing each inhalation and exhalation is a chance, a hope, a possibility.

"Whenever you have the chance," her letter concluded, "I would enjoy hearing what you are doing these days and knowing that you are safe and well. I think of you often with love."

* * *

The very long silence that followed was broken when I received a phone call from Melissa's mother, to tell me that Melissa had died on May 19, 2015. Because of my own physical limitations, I was not able to travel to Melissa's hometown community, located 24 miles from Philadelphia, where a memorial service for her was held. But 11 days after it had taken place, her mother mailed me a packet that contained the program of this event "in loving memory of Melissa, a woman of valor." It included the eulogies that were given by members of her family and by friends, in which were mentioned that I had been Melissa's "mentor" when she was a college student and that we had co-taught a seminar, and also a jump drive of the PowerPoint presentation put together for the service, in which there were two slides of Melissa and me. "Getting everything together [for you] was a true labor of love," Melissa's mother wrote in the note that accompanied the packet: "I wanted you to feel as if you were there. You meant so much to her. She talked about your friendship and how much you taught her. […] Perhaps I can come visit you some day and bring a copy of the manuscript we will put together of all her poetry. I know Melissa would love you to have it."

"I have a 'Melissa Goldstein file' that includes a number of her letters to me […… some of her poems], and other memorabilia, that I would like to share with you," I wrote in response:

And when you see it, if you feel you would like to have it, it would give me great happiness to pass it on to you so that you can be [its] keeper. […] This means that when you feel up to it, I would greatly welcome a visit from you. In the meanwhile, know that I am thinking of you and your family, mourning with you, and rejoicing with gratitude for the blessings that Melissa bestowed on me.

Chapter 17

WHAT I LEARNED ABOUT THE LANGUAGE OF SILENCE

The possibility of writing an essay about my relationship to religion occurred to me while I was drafting "Beyond Borders" and "On Being a Teacher," two of the essays included in this book. "Beyond Borders," which deals with the international and cross-cultural aspects of my work as a sociologist, contains an account of my participation in a center of sociological research that operated under the aegis of the episcopate of the Catholic Church in the Democratic Republic of Congo. And in the course of writing "On Being a Teacher," about my role as a teacher and my relationship with students, I was struck by the fact that many of the students with whom I have had close and lasting relations are attuned to what I would characterize as religiously resonant matters. They come from diverse religious backgrounds—Protestant, Catholic, Jewish, Islamic and Hindu among them. Some of them are religiously observant, some of them are not, and some regard themselves as "unreligious." Their differences notwithstanding, a significant number of them have this in common: through their work as health professionals and through the social scientific, historical or bioethical research they have conducted, they have been deeply involved with moral and human condition questions that bear on individual and social suffering and injustice associated with illness and medical care, and access to such care.

What influence might my own religious attitudes, values and beliefs have had on my career as a sociologist?, I wondered. For a while I seriously considered devoting an essay to this question, but I decided against it. In part I was deterred by how difficult I knew it would be for me to portray and explain, to myself as well as to others, my religious history and beliefs: those of a nonpracticing Jewess who was raised in a secularized Jewish family and who, like her parents, although strongly identified with her Jewish origins, was not learned in Judaism or a practicing member of a synagogue; who profoundly respected persons of faith in other religious traditions; and who, without being converted to Christianity, became involved in activities that linked her intellectually, professionally and personally to Catholicism. But the deep and fundamental reason for my decision not to write such an essay was my conviction that religion is a realm of my life and an essence of my being that can best be expressed in the language of silence rather than in the language of words.

* * *

In the Jewish setting in which I grew up, talking and writing were esteemed. Saying what you were thinking and feeling was viewed as a praiseworthy trait, and speaking eloquently and writing well were considered to be admirable gifts. It was not uncommon for silence to be experienced as worrisome or threatening because it was associated with a lack of ability to communicate with others—or an unwillingness to do so. The value that I accord to the importance and power of spoken and written words, to verbal expressiveness, and also to effectively speaking out in protest against unacceptable injustice, abuse and suffering have roots in these aspects of my background and upbringing.

It is only gradually in the course of my adult life that I have come to appreciate that silence is not simply an absence of words—a wordless vacuum—and that it can constitute a form of communication about matters that are too important to be expressed in words. I am reminded of an article written by the anthropologist Emiko Ohnuki-Tierney, in which she analyzes the deep meaning and great meaningfulness of what she calls "zero signifiers" in the Japanese language: "the absent pronouns in Japanese discourse, the concept of *ma* (empty space and time), and the concept of *mu* (nothingness)."[1] The evocatively insightful title that she gave her article is "The Power of Absence."[2]

---

[1] Emiko Ohnuki-Tierney, "The Power of Absence: Zero Signifiers and Their Transgressions," *L'Homme* 34, no. 130 (April–June 1994): 59–76, p. 61.

[2] I discussed this part of my essay with a former student, Katherine A. Mulhorn, PhD, who is now professor and chair in the Health Care Administration Department of Drexel University, and whose husband, Ayumu Yokoyama, is a chemical engineer of Japanese origins. After she, in turn, discussed the conceptions of silence in Ohnuki-Tierney's "The Power of Absence" article with him, he referred me to an article that he published about a workshop course he designed to help prepare engineering students deal with the culturally diverse origins of colleagues and clients in their future work (Ayumu Yokoyama, "An Innovative Method for Integrating a Diversity Workshop in a Chemical Engineering Course," *Chemical Engineering Education* 43, no. 1 (Winter 2009): 10–14). In this article he notes that "silence has many positive aspects in Asian culture, such as showing respect to superiors." In an email exchange with his wife that he intended her to share with me, Yokoyama explained that "the use of silence (*Ma*) in Japanese conversation show[s] respect to teachers, professors, or supervisors and also is used to provide enough time to reflect on what has been said, and to think about what to say next. Nothingness (*Mu*) is the state of mind that Zen meditation wants you to reach. With *Mu* you forget what is in

"Ultimately, worship and prayer have to do with silence rather than words," a professor of history who is also an Anglican priest once wrote to me. "And there is recognition, even in sacramental worship, that words are inadequate, and that symbolic actions speak louder than words." This was movingly apparent in the visit that Pope Francis made on July 29, 2016, to Auschwitz, the German Nazi concentration and extermination camp in Krakow, Poland. Before his arrival there, Pope Francis said he "would like to go to that place of horror without speeches, without crowds," to enter it alone, and to pray in silence—which he did. Rabbi David Rosen, the international director of interreligious affairs at the American Jewish Committee who accompanied him on this journey, commented that "in such a place, words are inadequate, and it's silence that becomes the ultimate expression of solidarity with the victims."[3]

* * *

I owe much of what I have learned and come to understand about the language and meaning of silence to the comportment, moral character and cultural traditions of four persons: one of my major teachers and two close, kin-like friends of "Old American" Protestant origins, and an intimate Catholic friend who grew up in the Flemish countryside of Belgium.

* * *

This is how and why the essay about my relationship to religion that I once contemplated writing became instead an essay about the significance of silence.

---

your mind and become aware of what is around you (your breathing, the wind, etc.) and become part of nature."

[3] Joanna Berendt, "Pope Francis, Visiting Auschwitz, Asks God for the 'Grace to Cry,'" *International New York Times.* www.nytimes.com/2016/07/30/world/europe/pope-francis-auschwitz.html.

Chapter 18

A BIOETHICS AWARD AND
A SURROGATE LECTURE

Let [me] congratulate you on being named the recipient of the Beecher
Award from the Hastings Center for 2015. […] [A]s the Chairman of
the nominating committee I have the honor and joy of notifying you first.
You will hear [officially] soon. We may not have had the opportunity of
much contact in recent years but I think I have known you for a longer
time than any colleague in the field, Dan Callahan included. I remember
visiting you at Smith when I was an undergrad at Harvard. And I also
remember your visit to Cleveland to our mutual friend Joanne King.
I hope the years have treated you with the kindness you deserve.

This email was sent to me by Willard (Will) Gaylin, Emeritus Clinical Professor
of Psychiatry at Columbia College of Physicians and Surgeons, who served on
Columbia's faculty as a training and supervising psychoanalyst for some thirty
years. In 1969, along with philosopher Daniel Callahan, he cofounded the
Hastings Center for Bioethics (initially called the Institute for Society, Ethics
and the Life Sciences), the first institution in the United States devoted to what
was then the nascent field of bioethics. The award to which he referred is the
center's Henry Knowles Beecher Award, which, in the words of its citation,
"recognizes individuals who have made a lifetime contribution to ethics and
the life sciences and whose careers have been devoted to excellence in scholarship, research, and ethical inquiry." Beecher was a distinguished physician-
anesthesiologist who, during the 1960s, the award's citation goes on to say,
"courageously shed light on ethically questionable practices in human subjects
research" and by these actions "helped give birth to the field of bioethics" in
which he "became one of its pioneers."[1]

As Will Gaylin's message suggested, my receipt of this award evoked aspects
of our long-ago personal and professional histories. We first met 70 years ago

---

[1] See his historic article in this regard: Henry K. Beecher, "Ethics and Clinical Research,"
New England Journal of Medicine 274 (June 16, 1966): 1354–60.

in my freshman year at Smith College, introduced by Joanne King, my closest college friend, whose hometown, like Will's, was Cleveland, Ohio. At that time, toward the close of World War II, Will was smartly dressed in the uniform of the Naval Reserve Officer Training Corps (NROTC) in which he was enrolled during his undergraduate years at Harvard. Our paths did not cross again until 1969, when the Hastings Center for Bioethics was founded. This was when I first met Daniel Callahan and became the only social scientist appointed to the center's initial board of directors.

* * *

Over the course of the ensuing development of the field of bioethics, I have been directly and indirectly involved in its unfolding, as a participant observer and as an observing participant. Prominent among my activities related to bioethics are membership on the President's Commission for the Study of Ethical Problems in Medicine and Biomedical and Behavioral Research (from 1979 to 1981) and on the editorial boards of a number of bioethics-centered publications, including the first edition of the *Encyclopedia of Bioethics*, published in 1978. Some of my own publications have been viewed by others involved in bioethics as pertinent to the field, particularly my book *Experiment Perilous* in which I ethnographically portrayed and analyzed the psychological and social stresses and moral dilemmas experienced by physicians and patients on a metabolic research ward; *The Courage to Fail* and *Spare Parts*, books about organ transplantation, the artificial kidney and the Jarvik-7 artificial heart that medical historian Judith Swazey and I coauthored; and another book by Judith Swazey and me, *Observing Bioethics,* based on our extensive interviewing of first- and second-generation figures associated with bioethics in the United States as well as our own firsthand experiences in the field.[2] The international scope of the sociology of medicine–relevant research I have done throughout my career has given me the opportunity to observe and follow how bioethics or its equivalents have developed in Belgium, France, China, Pakistan and South Africa.

---

[2] Renée C. Fox, *Experiment Perilous*. Renée C. Fox and Judith P. Swazey, *The Courage to Fail: A Social View of Organ Transplants and Dialysis* (Chicago: University of Chicago Press, 1974; revised paperback ed., 1978; republished with a new introduction by the authors, New Brunswick, NJ: Transaction Publishers, 2003). Renée C. Fox and Judith P. Swazey, *Spare Parts: Organ Replacement in American Society* (New York: Oxford University Press, 1991; paperback ed. with a new introduction by the authors, New Brunswick, NJ: Transaction Publishers, 2013). Renée C. Fox and Judith P. Swazey, *Observing Bioethics* (New York: Oxford University Press, 2008).

In lecturing, teaching and publishing about bioethics, I have consistently presented its import as extending beyond the development and establishment of an intellectual field that is primarily concerned with advances in biology and medicine, their relationship to illness and health, and their ethical concomitants. Although some of the value and belief questions with which bioethics has been preoccupied since its inception are expressed through the medium of medicine, I have contended that they are connected with broad and deep moral issues that are integral to what the illustrious French sociologist Émile Durkheim would have termed the collective conscience (*conscience collective*) of a society and its culture. At the same time, my macro-sociological perspective on the significance of bioethics has been a major source of my role as a constant critic of the field—above all, because of what I consider to be the deficiencies in its social, cultural and cross-cultural perspective on the questions and issues it examines.

Notwithstanding my persistent critique of bioethics, I have received two major bioethics awards. The Beecher Award was the second. The first was the Lifetime Achievement Award of the American Society for Bioethics and the Humanities (ASBH), which I received in 2007 at the society's annual meeting. I began my short acceptance talk for that award by saying that I hoped the assemblage would not think it impertinent for me to admit that I not only was surprised to be its recipient but found it somewhat ironic to be recognized in this way, given my recurrent criticisms of bioethics' shortcomings. I then proceeded to briefly outline the attributes of the bioethics I would like to see. The audience seemed to appreciate the self-mocking style in which I enumerated these attributes as much as—and probably more than—the ideas that my talk contained.[3]

The Beecher Award involved more elaborate preparations. To begin with, Mildred (Millie) Solomon, the president and CEO of the Hastings Center, had arranged for the 2015 award recipient to deliver a "featured event" kind of formal lecture at the American Society for Bioethics and Humanities' annual meeting. This lecture not only called for greater preparation on my part than was necessary for the casual talk I had given for my first bioethics award; it also required traveling to Houston, Texas, where the meeting was scheduled to be held. As I explained to Millie, although I was still in fundamentally good health at 87 years of age, my elderly body made such travel a daunting prospect. I proposed to her that rather than making the trip to Texas, I invite a distinguished member of the bioethics community to deliver the lecture that I would write, and to lead the discussion that I hoped it would evoke. She

---

[3] For a fuller account, see Fox, *In the Field*, pp. 329–30.

responded positively to this suggestion—all the more so when I told her that I had already spoken to Alexander Morgan Capron about whether he would be willing to assume this role, and that he had graciously consented to do so.

Alex Capron, an eminent jurist, a professor of law and medicine at the University of Southern California, and an internationally recognized expert in health policy and medical ethics, was the 2009 recipient of a Beecher Award. I came to know him during several early meetings of the Hastings Center and while we were both on the faculty of the University of Pennsylvania. My appreciation of the quality of his intellect and scholarship, his way of thought and his values was deepened by the part that he played in assisting Jay Katz (a professor of psychiatry and law at Yale University for a half-century) in writing the pioneering casebook *Experimentation with Human Beings*, and by his coauthorship with Katz of *Catastrophic Diseases: Who Decides What?*[4] In the memorial tribute that he paid to Katz at the time of Katz's death, Alex described Katz's contributions to the field of bioethics (for which Katz, too, had received a Beecher Award, in 1993) as being dedicated to "the vulnerable [...] the disadvantaged in our midst, those stripped of their rights and dignity"—including patients and research subjects—and to "the law's commitment to rational decision-making" with regard to their rights.[5] Alex has continued to espouse and express these values in the various arenas of his engagement with bioethics, including the important role he played as executive director of the President's Commission for the Study of Ethical Problems in Medicine and Biomedical and Behavioral Research, and in his extensive involvements in global aspects of bioethically relevant matters, including as director of Ethics, Trade, Human Rights and Health Law at the World Health Organization (WHO) in Geneva.[6] All of these attributes led me to ask Alex to stand in for me at the 2015 annual meeting of the ASBH, and I felt both grateful and honored when, without hesitation, he said that he would.

---

[4] Jay Katz, with the assistance of Alexander Morgan Capron and Eleanor Swift Glass, *Experimentation with Human Beings: The Authority of the Investigator, Subject, Profession, and State in the Human Experimentation Process* (New York: Russell Sage Foundation, 1972). Jay Katz and Alexander Morgan Capron, *Catastrophic Diseases: Who Decides What?* (New York: Russell Sage Foundation, 1975).

[5] Capron's remembrance was published in the *Hastings Center Report*: "Field Notes," *Hastings Center Report* 39, no. 1 (January–February 2009): c2.

[6] Capron served as executive director of the Commission from 1978 to 1983. I was able to observe him in action in this capacity during my term on the Commission. The Commission dealt with many topics and published such reports as *Defining Death*; *Protecting Human Subjects*; *Compensating for Research Injuries*; *Making Health Care Decisions*; *Splicing Life*; *Genetic Screening and Counseling*; *Deciding to Forego Life-Sustaining Treatment*; *Securing Access to Health Care*; and *Implementing Human Research Regulations*.

I shared several drafts of my lecture with Alex and incorporated the few small but significant editing suggestions that he made. Before the ASBH meeting, Millie Solomon and Bill Jeffway, the Hastings Center's director of marketing, communication and development, traveled to Philadelphia to videotape me in my study briefly introducing the lecture. The videotape would be played for the lecture's audience before Alex began speaking.

* * *

The text of my lecture begins with an affirmation of the more-than-medical social, cultural and moral significance that I attach to bioethics. Rather paradoxically, I continue, my appreciation of the larger meaning and ramifications of bioethics is a major source of the discontent that I also feel about the field, especially regarding the restricted nature of the empirical phenomena with which it is concerned and the body of principles and values that it applies to them.

Bioethics, I contend, seems to be inexorably preoccupied with the ethical concomitants of a relatively limited set of developments in biology, medicine and medical technology, such as those associated with genetics, neonatology, the replacement of human organs and life support techniques and treatments. Most of these developments bear on the beginning and the end of life, and on human personhood. Cross-cutting the field's concentration on these developments and issues has been its consistent foundational concern with research ethics, centered on human experimentation, especially on obtaining adequately informed voluntary consent from the human subjects on whom research is conducted.

I do not question the moral gravity of these matters, I go on to say in the lecture, or the seriousness with which bioethics has approached them. But I *am* troubled by the degree to which the field continues to pay more attention to the kinds of individual rights considerations that dealing with the human subjects of research and the care of dying persons entail than with issues that are associated with the common good, social solidarity, social justice and a global health ethic that recognizes that our individual health is linked to the community. In turn, I contend, this emphasis has contributed to bioethics paying relatively little attention to the implications of such situations as the plight of all the children in the world who suffer from hunger and chronic malnutrition (including in a society as affluent as the United States), as well as emerging, new and reemerging old infectious diseases, especially in the world's poorest countries—most recently, the devastating recent outbreak of Ebola in West Africa, and the failure of relevant national and international bodies to have adequately prepared for and responded to it.

My lecture proceeds to discuss some of the characteristics of bioethics, integral to its conceptual framework and to its ethos, that in my view have contributed to the field's relative nonengagement with grave societal and global issues like child hunger and epidemics of infectious diseases. The degree to which bioethics has been dominated by analytic philosophy, with its individualism-oriented emphasis on the principle of autonomy and its notion of a common morality which are more Western and American than universalistic in outlook, is one of these characteristics. Another is a wariness about the ethical relativism that might ensue from attaching too much importance to differences in social and cultural beliefs and values. I contend that this skew in bioethical thought is reinforced by what philosopher Onora O'Neill has characterized as the "tenuous interdisciplinarity" of the field,[7] and that, as a result, its institutionalized way of thought has not systematically drawn on the social sciences.

From here I move on in the lecture to muse about the virtual absence in the bioethics literature of a set of phenomena that are intrinsic to the practice of medicine—namely, medical uncertainty and iatrogenesis (the inadvertent adverse effects of medical and surgical actions that can, and often do occur notwithstanding the primary moral commandment to "do no harm" under which physicians practice medicine). I consider the inattentiveness of bioethics to these persistent phenomena that evoke painful ethical questions for physicians, their patients and their patients' families all the more perplexing, I say in the lecture, because of how salient I find them to be in the firsthand ethnographic research that I have conducted over the course of many years among medical students, physicians and patients, and how significant they are in the personal narratives, essays and memoirs of physicians.

(As I was writing this essay, for example, I was in the midst of reading a book titled *Do No Harm: Stories of Life, Death, and Brain Surgery* by neurosurgeon Henry Marsh, who characterizes surgery as "violence," albeit "controlled and altruistic," and who states with anguished candor that "few people outside medicine realize that what tortures doctors most is uncertainty, rather than the fact that they often deal with people who are about to die":

It is easy enough to let somebody die if one knows beyond doubt that they cannot be saved—if one is a decent doctor one will be sympathetic, but the situation is clear. This is life, and we all have to die sooner or later. It is when I do not know for certain whether I can help or not, or should help or not, that things become so difficult.

---

[7] Personal communication.

An infectious disease specialist physician also testifies about medical uncertainty, writing that, for her, "the hardest part of working with Ebola" at the height of its epidemic in Liberia "was not the physical exhaustion of working in personal protective equipment in the heat, the emotional impact of patients dying from a rapidly fatal disease, or personal concerns about becoming infected. It was, instead the lack of knowledge about Ebola, and not knowing if we could have done more to prevent people dying."[8])

I end the lecture by exhorting participants in the field of bioethics to more vigorously examine and discuss their ideas than they have characteristically done. In this connection, I invoke the example of the medical humanitarian organization Doctors Without Borders/Médecins Sans Frontières (MSF) that I have spent many years studying. One of MSF's most distinctive characteristics, I state, is what it calls its "culture of debate": "the vigorous and often combative self-reflection and self-criticism in which it continually engages."[9] If the members of an organization who are involved in frontline, often danger-fraught action have enough collective conviction and energy to continually participate in the self-searching examination of ideas—including of their principles—shouldn't the bioethics community, which exists and operates under more sheltered conditions, be capable of this, too? I challengingly ask. In conclusion, in the spirit of such debate, I invite those attending the Beecher lecture to question the validity of my critique of bioethics' shortcomings, and the soundness of my suggestions for the "betterment" of the field.

* * *

The session of the ASBH meeting at which Alex Capron presented my lecture was scheduled to take place on Saturday, October 24, from 2:00 p.m. to 3:30 p.m. Just before it began, I received a series of emails from a colleague and friend who was a member of the audience assembling for the lecture. "Your lecture is packed," he reported. "The biggest crowd I've seen at any talk here at ASBH." He emailed images of what he described as the "standing room only crowd," of the videotape of me presenting my introduction (which he labeled "Renée on the Big Screen"), and of Alex delivering the lecture from an impressive-looking podium.

---

[8] Henry Marsh, *Do No Harm*, p. 76. The American general and endocrine surgeon Atul Gawande, who I cite in my lecture, also characterizes surgery as an act of "calculated violence," carried out with a "righteous faith that it [is] somehow good for the [patient]." Atul Gawande, *Complications: A Surgeon's Notes on an Imperfect Science* (New York: Henry Holt, 2002), p. 16. Marsh, *Do No Harm*, p. 235. R. Burton, "Ebola: Experiences from the Field—Liberia," *South African Medical Journal* 105, no. 12 (2015): 1006–8, p. 1007.

[9] Renée C. Fox, *Doctors Without Borders*, p. 5.

Immediately after the lecture, Millie Solomon sent an exuberant email message to Alex, Bill Jeffway and me, saying: "Room was full, vibe was one of engagement, Alex was terrific, video was excellent, and many, many people came up to thank me. So now, I thank the three of you! Very well done!" She sent another email describing how well the event went to Dan Callahan, Will Gaylin and David Roscoe, chairman of the Hastings Center's Board, with a copy to me. Renée's "talk, the video and the whole session really was special," she wrote, "with the room full and people standing along the back wall [...]. Therefore am sharing the glow with you all and connecting you with Renée directly." David Roscoe responded by expressing "immense joy and great pride" in reading Millie's exchange. "Thanks for putting so much into what was truly a special event," he said in his email to me. "Dan and Will always have wanted the Beecher Award to be seen publicly as important to the community. There's no doubt that's the case now." Dan Callahan emailed me, too. Intermingled with his appreciative sentiments about how "glad" he was that my "event and lecture went so well," and what a "a great idea" it was to have Alex present my paper, was a pensive reference to the fact that "those of us from the old days are a dwindling group. [...] I basically don't travel much these days," he continued, "so have not been going to these or other meetings." Nonetheless, he affirmed, "despite a fair share of age problems [...] I continue to do well" and "have just finished one book, now in press, and another is almost done." ("A new book in press and another close to completion!!," I replied. "Congratulations! The ranks of our age group may be 'dwindling'—but *you* are not dwindling.")

It was Alex Capron's appraisal of how the lecture and whatever discussion it evoked had gone that I was especially eager to receive. Immediately after leaving the lecture, he emailed me a detailed account of what had transpired. "I wanted to reassure you," it began, "that although we were scheduled across from many other sessions which occupied the attention of many of your fans [...] (who expressed to me over the past couple of days their disappointment over missing the Beecher Lecture), the room was still packed. [...] Also your presence was very much felt, thanks to the wonderful video of your opening remarks."

Alex informed me that at the end of the lecture, he had told the audience that I was eager to have feedback from them that included challenges to the points I had made and the questions I had posed, along with relevant examples from their own experiences. Among what he termed "the points from the floor" that he conveyed to me were several that supported my characterization of discussion within US bioethics milieus as more "anemic" than the "culture of debate" and of self-criticism of MSF that I had described. An American member of the audience attributed this difference to the livelier cultural tradition of discussion in all settings, from the family table to the cafés to public forums, that she had observed while living in France. A French person in the audience agreed with her, and testified how much she enjoyed discussing with Dutch colleagues how shocked she was by the euthanasia of neonates in Holland, and with Irish colleagues the dismay she felt about the antiabortion principles that prevailed in Ireland.

Another commentator suggested that my portrayal of bioethics' hyper-individualism did not take sufficiently into account the "the big role" that the values of the common good, social solidarity and social justice play in the public health ethics branch of bioethics.

In the course of the allegations that I made in my lecture about bio-ethics' relative inattention to ethical issues associated with the ever-present incidence of infectious diseases and their epidemic-scale outbreaks, I mentioned that a major international clinical trial called START has recently provided definitive evidence that beginning antiretroviral therapy immediately after HIV is diagnosed would significantly improve the sur-vival of persons with HIV and lower the risk both of their developing opportunistic illnesses and of transmitting HIV to others. I went on to say that this ostensibly good news poses, on a massive scale, ethical problems about how to provide and equitably allocate antiretroviral medications, whose supply is already inadequate. One of the persons attending the lec-ture who was a member of the ethics review committee for the START trial in India, Cambodia and Vietnam, as it related to pediatric trials, responded to this part of the lecture by confirming that such a poten-tial crisis of good fortune did indeed exist in those settings—one that in her opinion was particularly acute with regard to the applicability of its findings to the early treatment of children.

And after he left the lecture, Alex reported to me, "another listener expressed surprise" to him personally about my "failure to mention the effects of persistent racism, in society and in the health care system, as a major ethical issue about which bioethics has said relatively little." "To which I would add a question," Alex wrote to me: "Does this reflect, in part, the relative paucity of people of color within bioethics?"

"You would have been very gratified," Alex concluded, "to see how well your remarks were received, notwithstanding their having been delivered by a […] surrogate. For me, it was a great honor to have been entrusted with this duty." He "signed off" on a humorous note. "I now have the singular distinc-tion of having 'presented' two Beecher lectures!" he wrote, self-deprecatingly referring to his Beecher award in 2009.

* * *

As I reflect on the lecture I prepared for the award ceremony, I reach the conclusion that it is as unlikely that my lecture will have an enduring effect as it is that I will be the recipient of a *third* bioethical *lifetime* award (if any other such awards exist!).[10]

----

[10] On the 50th anniversary of the publication of Henry Beecher's landmark whistle-blowing article in *The New England Journal of Medicine* about ethical abuses in clinical research, the journal *Perspectives in Biology and Medicine* devoted a special issue in 2016 to "the historical significance and continuing legacy" of that article. The text of my Beecher lecture, with the title "Moving Bioethics Toward Its Better Self: A Sociologist's Perspective," is included.

EPILOGUE

On June 27, 2017, as he celebrated with the assembled cardinals the 25th anniversary of his ordination as a bishop, Pope Francis took as his text a reading from the book of Genesis about God's call to Abraham when Abraham was about the same age as the Pope—who was then 80 years old. When God called Abraham, he was "about to enter retirement, retirement to rest." Abraham was "an elderly man, with the burden of old age, [...] old age that brings aches and pains, illness." But God told him to "Rise, go, go!" as though he were a young man, as if he "were a scout: Go! Look and hope." "This Word of God is also for us, who are of an age similar to that of Abraham," the Pope told the cardinals. "The Lord tells us that our history is still open: it is open until the end; it is open with a mission. And he indicates our mission with these three imperatives: "Rise! Look! Hope!" The Pope concluded, "We are grandfathers [...] called to dream and to give our dream to today's young people: they need it. Because they will draw from our dreams the power to prophecy and carry out their task."[1]

As this collection of essays indicates, notwithstanding the limitations and frailties to which I am now subject, I continue to have a rich and mentally vigorous life as a sociologist who is still actively engaged in participant observation. I have found much that is sociologically interesting and potentially significant in settings as close at hand as the apartment building where I live, and the streets surrounding it. What is more, through the far-reaching network of colleagues, former students, and friends with whom I am connected and communicate, I am continually in contact with the multiple American, European, African and Asian contexts in which I previously conducted research, and with events and developments of import that are occurring in those settings.

---

[1] "Eucharistic Concelebration with the Cardinals Resident in Rome on the Occasion of the 25th Anniversary of the Episcopal Ordination of the Holy Father, Homily of His Holiness Pope Francis, Pauline Chapel, June 27, 2017." https://w2.vatican.va/content/francesco/en/homilies/2017/documents/papafrancesco_20170627_xxvordinazepiscopale-papafrancesco.html.

As a retired "emerita" professor, I no longer do classroom teaching. I would not be physically capable of commuting to a college or university campus for that purpose. And yet, I feel like a teacher, am still viewed as one, and have opportunities to fulfill that role from inside the confines of my apartment. I am in touch with a surprisingly large number of persons whom I once taught, stretching all the way back to my initial years as a faculty member at Barnard College from 1955 to 1966. My former students keep me abreast of their personal, familial and professional news, and ask for my advice concerning professional plans and decisions they are contemplating, and for recommendations on their behalf in this connection. In growing numbers, I hear from young professionals as well as undergraduate and graduate students I have not previously taught who are working on projects relevant to my publications. Both former and new students visit me for face-to-face conversations.

Over the course of the years that I have been writing these essays, I have progressed from the eighth decade of my life to the threshold of the ninth. I would be falsifying what these elderly years are like if I ended this book with an unequivocal Pollyannaish affirmation about them. In April 2016, I unpredictably and inexplicably fell in my kitchen. This resulted in several fractured ribs and two weeks in a rehabilitation center. Although my ribs have healed, and I have resumed my daily round in my apartment, I am experiencing some signs of physical deconditioning and of increased anxiety about my sense of balance and the possibility of falling again. In addition, I have developed age-related macular degeneration in my left eye. It is the leading cause of vision loss among older Americans. Mine is the so-called wet kind. It is not curable, but it is being treated by periodic injections directly into the eye of a drug called *Lucentis*.

The disquietude I am currently experiencing is not confined to personal concern about my physical well-being and fortitude. It includes my angst about the occurrence and implications of some of the kinds of national, international and global events with which I have dealt in these essays. But as I have chronicled, the questing, observation, reflection and teaching in which I am still engaged, and the extensive, vibrant network of which I am a part, leaven these years, infuse them with purpose and meaning, and embolden me to have hope for the future that will extend beyond my lifetime.

For all this, I am very grateful.

www.ingramcontent.com/pod-product-compliance
Lightning Source LLC
Chambersburg PA
CBHW022356280326
41935CB00007B/206